Unconscious Knowing and Other Essays in Psycho-Philosophical Analysis

International Perspectives in Philosophy and Psychiatry

Series editors: KWM (Bill) Fulford, Katherine Morris, John Z Sadler, and Giovanni Stanghellini

Volumes in the series:

Unconscious Knowing and Other Essays in Psycho-Philosophical Analysis

Linda A.W. Brakel

Departments of Philosophy and Psychiatry

The University of Michigan

Ann Arbor, Michigan

USA

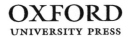

OXFORD

UNIVERSITY PRESS

OXFORD
UNIVERSITY PRESS

Great Clarendon Street, Oxford OX2 6DP

Oxford University Press is a department of the University of Oxford.
It furthers the University's objective of excellence in research, scholarship,
and education by publishing worldwide in

Oxford New York

Auckland Cape Town Dar es Salaam Hong Kong Karachi
Kuala Lumpur Madrid Melbourne Mexico City Nairobi
New Delhi Shanghai Taipei Toronto

With offices in

Argentina Austria Brazil Chile Czech Republic France Greece
Guatemala Hungary Italy Japan Poland Portugal Singapore
South Korea Switzerland Thailand Turkey Ukraine Vietnam

Oxford is a registered trade mark of Oxford University Press
in the UK and in certain other countries

Published in the United States
by Oxford University Press Inc., New York

British Library Cataloguing in Publication Data
Data available

Library of Congress Cataloging in Publication Data
Data available

Typeset by Glyph International, Bangalore, India
Printed in Great Britain
on acid-free paper by
MPG Books Group, Bodmin and King's Lynn

ISBN 978–0–19–958147–4

10 9 8 7 6 5 4 3 2 1

To my parents, Paula and Walter Wimer;
and to my earliest intellectual forebears,
Uncles Ernie and Kurt Wimer

Permissions Granted

I thank the following publishing agencies and societies for their kind permission to publish, in the present volume, revised versions of works previously published and for illustrations previously published. These are:

The American Psychoanalytic Association for Fig 2.2, page 33 of the current volume. This figure first appeared in an article whose citation is as follows: **Brakel, LAW** (1993). 'Shall drawing become part of free association: a proposal for a modification in psychoanalytic technique'. *Journal of the American Psychoanalytic Association*, **41**, 359–394. The figure appeared as 'Figure 2' on page 364.

The Johns Hopkins University Press, acknowledged and thanked for their kind permission for publishing here:

1. Chapter 5, adapted from an article: **Brakel, LAW** (2007). 'The placebo effect: Can psychoanalytic theory explain the phenomenon?' Copyright © 2007 The Johns Hopkins University Press. This article first appeared in *American Imago*, **64**, Issue 2, Summer, 2007, 273–281; and

2. Chapter 2, adapted from an article: **Brakel, LAW** (2008). 'Knowledge and Belief: psychoanalytic evidence in support of a radical epistemic view.' Copyright © 2008 The Johns Hopkins University Press. This article first appeared in *American Imago*, **65**, Issue 3, Fall, 2008, 427–471.

Preface

Aims

This book is a thoroughly interdisciplinary project involving psychoanalytic theory and philosophy—specifically the philosophy of mind, action, science, and metaphysics. In each chapter, I describe a particular problem that has long been of interest to philosophers and psychoanalysts (theorists and practitioners). My initial aim is to solve the puzzles presented—all to the good if I can do so in novel ways. However, the book has two other aims as well. First, to demonstrate that by using concepts and tools both from philosophy and psychoanalysis the problems themselves can be more deeply examined and thereby appreciated. Second, to establish that these interdisciplinary investigations provide the exciting potential to enhance aspects of theory in both disciplines. Finally, there is a matter that is not an aim of the book so much as a hope: namely, that others will find this approach sufficiently interesting that they will develop specific criteria for identifying future topics that would benefit from a psycho–philosophical analysis.

Acknowledgments

I thank those at Oxford (UK) University Press, particularly my editors, Martin Baum, for allowing this project to take flight at all, and Charlotte Green, for helping the book take shape at each stage. For providing a forum for discussing these ideas, I thank Randolph M. Nesse and the Wednesday Research Lab Group at the University of Michigan. For reviewing and commenting on earlier drafts of various chapters, I thank Allan Gibbard, Jim Joyce, Daniel Moerman, Jack Novick, Peter Rudnytsky, and Timothy Williamson. Then there are two others who, while they each also reviewed and commented on an early version of a chapter, did much more both emotionally and intellectually. Therefore, I express my gratitude to David Velleman, and especially to my husband (best friend and first critic), Arthur Brakel.

Contents

Part I

Introduction

Chapter 1

Introduction

Introduction

Unconscious Knowing and Other Essays in Psycho-Philosophical Analysis, although in no way a sequel to *Philosophy, Psychoanalysis, and the A-Rational Mind* (Oxford, 2009), presents further investigations at the intersection(s) of analytic philosophy and psychoanalytic theory. In that earlier volume I held that psychoanalysis, despite its elegant theory, would benefit from philosophical sharpening of many of its concepts; and that the philosophy of mind could and should expand its domain of interest to include the unconscious and a-rational mind. In the current work I take a further step, suggesting that there are important topics that cannot be well understood unless viewed from the interdisciplinary perspective of psychoanalytic theory and particular branches of philosophy (mind, action, epistemology, metaphysics, science, etc.). Moreover, there are longstanding puzzles in both fields that will more readily reveal solutions if tools from both disciplines are employed.

The current collection is more focused than my earlier book as well as more diverse. Whereas *Philosophy, Psychoanalysis, and the A-Rational Mind* was anchored in addressing problems directly related to the general psychoanalytic theory of mind, and sought to provide a-rational thought with a philosophical grounding, *Unconscious Knowing and Other Essays in Psycho-Philosophical Analysis* considers four distinct areas in depth, united only by their being potentially of interest both to philosophers of various types and psychoanalytic theorists and clinicians. I say 'potentially' because academics in related disciplines are increasingly losing the will, and with that the ability, to communicate about matters of mutual and vital concern. For example, philosophers and psychoanalysts have important things to say about 'mind,' 'concept,' 'category,' 'unconscious,' 'non-conscious,' 'rational,' 'irrational,' 'belief,' 'knowledge,' 'phantasy,' 'self,' and 'agent'; yet the psychoanalytic and philosophical literatures bearing on these issues are very separate, save for superficial, or even worse, tendentious cross-referencing. Ideally, this volume will play a part toward reversing that trend by marshalling concepts, contents, and forms drawn both from academic philosophy and psychoanalysis (clinical and theoretical) in addressing the four topics.

Following this Introduction, Chapter 2, 'Unconscious knowing: Psychoanalytic evidence in support of a radical epistemic view,' will take up the first of the four topics—unconscious knowledge. The very idea of unconscious knowledge leads immediately to considerations of the broader issue of knowledge versus belief. That there can be unconscious knowledge at all and the recognition of the great importance of unconscious knowing in mental life, together constitute one of the most basic assumptions of psychoanalytic theory. However, from the philosophical viewpoint most modern epistemologists have contended that belief, rather than knowledge, is the most fundamental mental attitude. The chapter begins with Timothy Williamson's (2000) account, which shifts knowledge back to the foundational center. Much space in the chapter is devoted to providing support for this radical knowledge-centered view, both from clinical psychoanalytic data, and research findings on unconscious processes, as well as from other research cognate to psychoanalytic presuppositions. I use a variety of comparisons between belief and knowledge, both conscious and unconscious, to make the case.

Chapter 3, 'The limits of rationality: Vagueness, a case study' is obviously about vagueness. Not so obviously, however, Chapter 3 presents a discovery. When philosophers deal with the concept of vagueness (which is itself a vague concept), they do so with much precision and rationality. And yet, often emerging from work on this topic are very interesting philosophical accounts, many of which bear a surprising resemblance to the contentful notions held by all manner of primary process a-rational thinkers. Once the power and scope of a-rationality is seen in this unusual context, promising implications for greater understanding of the deep nature of our cognitive system(s) follow, as do intriguing ontological speculations regarding the constitution of the (our?) world. This chapter provides much background both about a-rationality and vagueness, and it highlights their similarity.

Agency is the main issue addressed in Chapter 4, 'Agency: "me"-ness in action.' Agency is a topic of interest both to philosophers of action and to psychoanalysts. In this chapter, I advance the idea that, in most clinical psychoanalyses, questions of agency are far more important than psychoanalytic theoreticians and clinicians have realized. Parallel with this, I find that agency also figures prominently in a vexing philosophical problem, characterized by the following question: When I am concerned about my continued survival, just what is the nature of the 'me' with which I am concerned? It is one's agency, I argue, that constitutes my 'me'-ness. The chapter goes on to develop an account of agency as singular, directly related to one's willingness to act, and characterized by behaviors that can answer 'why' questions of both a psychological and biological sort.

Chapter 5 is titled 'The placebo effect: Psychoanalytic theory can help explain the phenomenon.' This chapter is perhaps less complicated than the others in its structure. I review and describe the placebo effect and outline some of the mechanisms, known and speculated, contributing to its cause. Further, I argue that underlying the placebo effect are two processes very much tied to psychoanalysis: positive transference and positive conditioning. The former *is* a psychoanalytic concept. The latter owes its connection to psychoanalysis to the a-rational primary process operations that are essential to aspects of classical conditioning including, most importantly, the generalizations necessary to produce conditioned stimuli and conditioned responses. Once this connection is demonstrated, the chapter's main assertion can be made clear. The roles of conditioning and positive transference are central to the placebo effect, and as each of these processes is constituted by psychoanalytic concepts, psychoanalytic concepts can indeed help explain the placebo effect.

The final chapter, Chapter 6, 'Explanations and Conclusions' takes a particular slant on all of the work presented in this volume. Here, I offer not so much an assessment of whether the interdisciplinary approach has been successful, but instead an exploration of the sorts of explanations each of these chapters has offered. Explanations about the phenomena of explanations are also an important part of this last chapter. The explanatory contributions of Chapters 2, 3, and 4 are less scientific, and therefore less ambitious than what I attempt in Chapter 5. Thus characterizing the types of explanations in Chapters 2, 3, and 4 is brief. I advance a far more extensive analysis of the nature of the explanation provided in the placebo chapter. I conclude Chapter 6 with assessments of the book as a whole.

A few general remarks: each chapter has its own blend of philosophy and psychoanalytic theory; with philosophy of mind, action, science, epistemology, and metaphysics all represented in various sections of the volume. Further, each chapter is written so that it can be read alone. This, and the fact that the book is intended to be understandable both to philosophers with little psychoanalytic knowledge and to psychoanalysts with interest in philosophy but little or no formal training in that field, necessitates that a great amount of background material be included in most chapters, particularly the early ones.[1] Admittedly, this does not usually make for the most fluid reading. I hope that the tradeoff yielding greater and more widespread comprehension is worth the

---

[1] Later chapters do make reference to the background material in the earlier ones.

effort so that, in the end, this work at the intersection of these ever-fascinating philosophical and psychoanalytic topics will spark further investigations.

References

Brakel, LAW (2009). *Philosophy, Psychoanalysis, and the A-Rational Mind.* Oxford, Oxford University Press.

Williamson, T (2000). *Knowledge and Its Limits.* Oxford, Oxford University Press.

Part II

Unconscious knowing

Epistemology, philosophy of mind

Chapter 2

Unconscious knowing: Psychoanalytic evidence in support of a radical epistemic view[1]

Introduction

In most standard contemporary work in philosophy of mind and epistemology, *knowledge* is considered some form of *true belief*. (See Armstrong 1973, p.137; Margolis 1973, p.3; Goldman 1975, p.111; and also Williamson 2000, p.2, who emphatically does not share this view but notes it historically.) Until the publication of the Gettier cases (Gettier 1963) this issue seemed largely settled with *justified true belief* regarded as the type of belief that simply *was* knowledge. (See Danto 1968, p.73; Shope 1983, pp.10–11.) After Edmund Gettier (1963) presented cases in which even justified true belief could not suffice for knowledge,[2] the status of justified true belief *as* knowledge did

---

[1] This chapter is a revised version of an earlier article: Brakel, LAW (2008). Knowledge and belief: psychoanalytic evidence in support of a radical epistemic view, *American Imago*, 65: 427–471.

[2] The purpose of this long footnote is to illustrate: a) justified true beliefs that seem to constitute knowledge, b) justified true beliefs that do not constitute knowledge (Gettier-like cases), c) unjustified true beliefs, and d) justified false beliefs. To begin with, take the following five facts as true: 1) It is Friday evening at 5 pm. 2) Our front doorbell is broken. 3) Vic, a punctual visitor at 5 pm each day, arrives on this particular Friday at 5 pm and presses the broken doorbell, but does not knock on the door. 4) Meanwhile, at 5 pm I hear what sounds to be a knock on the door. 5) Also, there has been a strong wind blowing intermittently for hours, and at 5 pm a medium-sized tree branch hits our front door just as Vic is 'ringing' the broken doorbell. So with these in mind, here is a) an example of a simple justified true belief that seems consistent with knowledge: I have the justified true belief/knowledge that since the doorbell does not work, some other sound (like a knock) will be needed to signal a visitor's presence. Now, for b) a Gettier-like case, where justified true beliefs do not constitute knowledge: On the basis of the 'knock' sound at 5 pm, I believe that someone is at the door, especially as I am expecting Vic. Although this was a justified and true belief—justified as it is rational to think that when doorbells are broken

indeed change. But, interestingly, the quest to explain knowledge in terms of belief did not change. Belief continued to be held among the conditions necessary, but alas not sufficient for knowledge (Margolis 1973, p.3; Goldman 1975, pp.111–112). Thus, according to Timothy Williamson (2000), for the last four decades many epistemologists 'have expended vast efforts attempting to state exactly what kind of true belief knowledge is' (p.2).[3] Williamson holds that philosophers of mind, similarly, 'marginalize the category of knowledge' insofar as 'belief is what matters for the understanding of the mind'—belief being the mental attitude that aims at the truth, and truth obtaining only when the truth conditions of the belief match those of the world (p.2).[4] For these philosophers too then, knowledge not only entails belief but is also 'merely a peculiar kind of true belief' (p.2), one requiring at least two additions to the mental state of belief—first, truth, as is needed also for true belief, and then

people will knock to signal their arrival, and that knocking makes the type of knock-sound I heard; and true in that Vic truly was at the door at 5 pm—still, I cannot be said to have had knowledge of Vic being at the door at 5 pm, because the appropriate causal chain did not figure into my justified true belief. I believed Vic was at the door due to what turns out to have been the false belief that Vic had knocked on the door when really the 'knock' was the sound of the branch banging against the door. c) An unjustified true belief is as follows: My husband, Art, was daydreaming at 5 pm that someone was at the door. On this a-rational basis he believed that someone was at the door. Since there was a visitor at 5 pm—this turned out to be a true belief. However, this belief was true only by accident; Art arrived at it without sufficiently justifiable reasons. Finally to illustrate d) a justified false belief, let us change one of the facts above. It is still Friday at 5 pm, but Vic does not arrive until 5:30 pm. At 5 pm when I heard the knocking sound, expecting Vic at 5 pm, I had the justified belief that it was Vic. As in the Gettier-like case above (example b), the knocking sound was really the branch hitting the door; but this time Vic was not yet present. My belief that it was someone at the door was equally justified, but under these circumstances it was false.

[3] Williamson (2000) maintains that some have insisted 'that knowledge *is* justified true belief on an understanding of "justified" strong enough to exclude Gettier cases but weak enough to include everyday empirical knowledge' (p.4). This is a view Williamson finds circular, lacking in a standard for justification sufficiently independent of knowledge.

[4] Because beliefs (by definition) are those cognitive attitudes that aim at the truth, they are attitudes regulated by evidence (See, e.g., Velleman 2000, p.16). Thus if Ari holds a belief B with the content that X is T, and this content is shown to Ari to be false, then Ari can no longer hold B as a belief. Ari can still have the content that X is T in other cognitive attitudes, e.g., as a supposition or a phantasy, but no longer as a belief.

Note that in this chapter (and volume) religious and cultural 'beliefs,' and the class of cognitive attitudes I have termed 'neurotic-beliefs' (Brakel 2001, 2009), will not be taken up as beliefs as none of these are evidence sensitive. Neurotic-beliefs will be discussed more fully much later in this chapter and in various places throughout this volume. (See also footnote 13, and the subsection on 'Anti-luminosity' in this chapter.)

'other more elusive features' (p.3).[5] Thus both for epistemologists—attempting to specify the essence of knowledge and belief—and for philosophers of mind, attempting to gain knowledge of the mind, belief is maintained as the foundational attitude, conceptually prior to knowledge.

Does this have to be the case? Or, are there arguments and evidence for the reverse: That it is knowledge that comes first, conceptually and ontologically, with belief dependent on knowledge, and not vice versa? In other words, what if the standard view has it backwards; that it is belief (justified or not; true or not) that is always predicated on, built upon, and entailing knowledge? What would be implied? In this chapter, I will advance this 'radical view,' presenting data both from psychoanalysis and cognitive neuropsychology to support philosophical arguments (owing largely to Williamson 2000, but including a few others) for this position. In so doing I hope not only to provide converging evidence for the radical view, but also to illustrate the strength of interdisciplinary approaches to questions that can only be properly located at an interface between or among disciplines—in this case epistemology, psychoanalytic theory, cognitive neuropsychology, and philosophy of mind.

So to begin I will present a case in which the agent in question has much knowledge but amazingly no belief at all about what he knows. This case comprises the section called 'Knowing without seeing or believing: A very striking negative hallucination' which follows immediately below. The subsequent sections are: 'Differences between knowledge (knowing) and belief (believing)'; 'Similarities between knowledge (knowing) and belief (believing)'; 'First- and second-order knowledge and belief: Believing what one knows, knowledge without belief'; 'Unconscious knowledge and unconscious belief'; 'The priority of knowledge'; and finally 'Psychoanalysis and the priority of knowledge.' Indeed, there is much ground to cover. Thus without further introduction, here is the clinical backbone of this chapter, the negative hallucination.

Knowing without seeing or believing: A very striking negative hallucination

Many years ago when I was a Resident in Psychiatry, and consequently often sleep deprived, I fell asleep for about 10 seconds during a session with a patient (Dr. N) in psychoanalytic psychotherapy. He had to have been aware of my

---

[5] When a concept is a conjunction of two concepts it is not as foundational as the conjuncts. For example, the concept 'striped shirt' is a conjunction of the concepts 'shirt' and 'striped,' both of which are more fundamental than striped shirt. Clearly, for the philosophers under discussion, 'knowledge' is conjunctive and not as fundamental as 'belief,' one of its conjuncts.

closed eyes and nodding head, as we faced each other directly and our chairs were no more than 6 feet apart. Through the rest of that session, as I had been taught to do, I listened and looked carefully for any sign of his reaction, direct or derivative. However, there were no allusions to careless doctors, sleepy people, inappropriate activities, consumers not getting what they pay for, inattentive women, etc., and no physical changes in Dr. N—not in that session.

However, at the start of our next meeting Dr. N recounted the following dream: 'I (Dr. N) fell asleep in our session. You (Dr. B) didn't seem to notice.' He added that, 'there was not much feeling in the dream.' I told Dr. N that his dream must be a reaction to his noticing my having fallen asleep in front of him during our previous session. He reacted as if I were crazy, saying with much animation: 'What are you talking about? You didn't fall asleep here last time! If you had, I'd be really furious.' Now, *I* was incredulous. It seemed impossible that he had not seen me. I was right in his line of vision, the lighting was not unusual, and certainly I was a salient stimulus object. True, he had, in his brief associations, provided a 'reason' for not-seeing me—he would be furious with me; and Dr. N was a man who was quite afraid that he could not adequately control his rage. But how could he not have had full conscious awareness of something that he recaptured so accurately in his dream? Obviously (to me) the thin disguise of reversing our roles did not obscure the contents—identical in dream and waking life—that one person, A, fell asleep right in front of the other person, B; yet Person B had not seemed to notice.

Dr. N, in a) not observing my falling asleep, b) dreaming the unseen content in thin disguise, and c) not recapturing the percept, had had an instance of what is known as a negative hallucination. This particular psychological event had pivotal psychoanalytic significance in two ways: 1) Clinically, Dr. N was forced to confront the fact that I had fallen asleep in his session and, that despite his robust defensive efforts to feel very little, both in reality and in the dream, he was in fact furious. 2) Theoretically, the event was instructive regarding the limits of psychoanalytic explanation. *Why* my patient would have had a negative hallucination given his conflicts and character—this type of question could (and can) be adequately addressed in terms of psychoanalytic clinical theory.[6] But the *how*—how he could not-see something he had to

---

6 Note too, that negative hallucinations do take place normally, or at least as part of the psychopathology of everyday life. Here is an example. One day my husband and I were walking in town when a man passed very close to us going the other way. The man looked familiar to me but I could not place him. I asked my husband, who replied, 'what man?' Immediately thereafter, my husband began to sing a refrain from a Simon and Garfunkel song titled 'So Long, Frank Lloyd Wright.' The refrain in question had the words,

have seen—this type of question remains unanswerable by psychoanalytic theory alone. Yet once one observes that the responses of subjects in subliminal experiments are structurally analogous to those of patients with negative hallucinations (see Brakel 1989), answers to questions of this sort can begin to be addressed through research into the processing of subliminal stimuli. The sort of research involved—cognitive and neuropsychological—is a cognate to, but is outside and independent of psychoanalysis.[7]

Beyond their psychoanalytic clinical and theoretical implications, for our present purposes it is the philosophical importance of negative hallucinations that is of greatest interest. Negative hallucinations can help illuminate aspects of the complex interrelationships among seeing, not-seeing, believing, and knowing—these last two being of special relevance here. Dr. N claimed not to have seen me fall asleep. Although he ultimately did not doubt my account of what transpired—and his own dream provided confirming evidence—he never did recapture the experience of having seen me nod-off right in front of him. Consequently, before my explanation, Dr. N had *no beliefs* at all about the incident he did not see. But would it be plausible or even coherent to say that he had *no knowledge* of it? Given his dream, and that my comments about my falling asleep followed his dream report, defending the position that he lacked knowledge would be difficult. For if indeed he had no knowledge of my sleeping, how would he have dreamed and reported the particular dream contents he did, given that they mirrored so precisely what happened? Dr. N had *knowledge*, more specifically *unconscious knowledge*, of the contents in question without the conscious experience of seeing anything, and without any sort of belief, justified or not, true or false, about the matter. This case suggests that knowledge is dependent neither on beliefs nor on seeing. Dr. N did not see anything about my sleeping; he had no beliefs about it; and yet, as his dream showed, he knew all about it, *unconsciously*.[8]

'architects may come and architects may go.' I then knew that the man who had passed was our architect's assistant. When I told my husband, he still believed he had seen no one; though of course he believed my account.

[7] Later in the chapter I shall offer more examples from these areas. See the section 'First- and second-order knowledge and belief: believing what one knows and knowing without beliefs.'

[8] Furthermore, the dream content suggests that he unconsciously knew the further fact that he experienced himself as not having consciously noticed my falling asleep because, in the dream, I do not notice his having fallen asleep.

Could Dr. N have had an unconscious belief instead of, or in addition to, his unconscious knowledge? I think not; although the argument against this view will be not be developed until later in the chapter, in the section, 'Unconscious knowledge/unconscious belief.'

Dr. N's negative hallucination clearly raises a number of issues concerning knowledge and belief at the intersection of philosophy of mind, epistemology, and psychoanalysis. The case certainly seems to lend support to the radical view that knowledge, rather than belief, is the more fundamental and foundational mental state. Let us proceed with our exploration of the relations between belief and knowledge to see if that view holds up.

Differences between knowledge (knowing) and belief (believing)

The relations between knowledge (knowing) and belief (believing) are of central import in determining whether or not knowledge is merely a type of true belief. If knowledge is only some type of true belief, on this ground, belief should be considered foundational and conceptually prior to knowledge. The opposite case, that for knowledge being prior to belief, must also rely on the relations between these two mental states. Hence, in this section, the differences between knowledge and belief are explored, and in the section that follows I explore their similarities.

General differences

To introduce the notion of a significant difference between knowledge and belief, let me start with H. A. Pritchard (1950), a philosopher who was so convinced of important general differences, that he asserted 'dogmatically...[and without]...offer of reasons' (p.87) the following:

> Knowing and believing differ in kind...Their difference in kind is not that of species and genus, like that of a red colour and a colour [simpliciter]. To know is not to have a belief of a special kind, differing from beliefs of other kinds; and no improvement in a belief and no increase in the feeling of conviction which it implies will convert it into knowledge. Nor is their difference that of being two species of a general genus. It is not that there is a general kind of activity...which admits of two kinds, the better of which is knowing and the worse believing (pp.87–88).

Another philosopher, J.J. Macintosh (1979–80) does offer an interesting *reductio ad absurdum* type of argument for the general difference. He starts with the counterargument that the mental state of knowing really is just the mental state of believing because when we find out that what we thought we knew is wrong, 'what we replace it with is not a claim that we used to know (though we now no longer do) but rather a claim that we used to *believe*, though we now no longer do. But our mental state was what it was...all along: And if we are now correct in speaking of ourselves as having a *belief*, then a belief it also was [before]' (p.171). However, Macintosh continues, if knowing is thereby accepted as a kind of believing '...by the same argument we can show that seeing is a kind *of*...hallucinating; that being awake is a kind *of*... dreaming, and so on' (p.180).

Both philosophers allude to what is probably the most important general difference between knowledge and belief, and certainly the most obvious: Namely, that whereas what is believed can be either true or false, what is known is either true or it is not knowledge. This is reflected in Robert Shope's (1983) statement, 'We may say that what is false is what we believed (but not what we knew)' (p.173). One way of understanding this difference is to suggest that a strictly internalist[9] account of knowledge as a mental state cannot possibly work, whereas for belief such an account could suffice.[10] Thus, on the internalist view, all that is needed to have identical beliefs about X are identical *internal* mental/brain states. So given whatever is needed neurologically to qualify as identical mental/brain states, S's belief that 'p is q' when p *is* q, is identical to S's belief that 'p is q' when p *is not* q. In other words, S's belief that 'that ball is in that corner' when the ball is there in that corner, is identical to S's belief that 'that ball is in that corner' when someone (unbeknownst to S) has moved the ball from the corner. This clearly will not work for knowledge. S's knowledge that 'p is q' when p *is* q, cannot be identical to S's ~knowledge[11] that 'p is q' when p *is not* q. While S can know that 'that ball is in that corner' when the ball is there, S cannot *know* that 'that ball is in that corner' when it is not. Facts about the world, facts *external* to S's brain states, must contribute to the mental state of knowledge.

Another general difference between knowledge and belief, widely agreed upon, is that whereas there are degrees of belief, there can be no degrees of knowledge. Regarding knowledge as a psychological state, Joseph Margolis (1973) states, 'that someone knows that p is an all-or-nothing affair; this is not true...of such psychological states as beliefs: One may half-believe, half-disbelieve' (p.35). Roderick Chisolm (1957) puts it like this: 'A man can be said to believe firmly, or reluctantly or hesitantly, but no one can be said to know firmly, reluctantly or hesitantly' (p.18). Relatedly, one can even evaluate beliefs, but not knowledge, as 'silly or sensible; or as mature versus childlike' (Shope 1983, p.176). (See also Ring 1977, p.57 for a similar account of the general differences.)

---

[9] Internalism will be briefly explained just below.

[10] But see the next section 'Similarities between knowledge (knowing) and belief (believing)' for the view that a strictly internalist account cannot work for belief either.

[11] The symbol ~ is used to indicate 'not.'

Owing to this difference between them, although both beliefs and knowledge are regulated by truth conditions in the world and therefore sensitive to evidence, beliefs are much more apt to be changed given new evidence whereas knowledge is much more stable and sturdy. This is a point made by Norman Malcolm (1952, p.80), Arthur Danto (1968, p.108) who cites Malcolm, and Williamson (2000, pp.7–8, 62–63) who states: 'Although knowing is not invulnerable to destruction by later evidence, its nature is to be robust in that respect. Stubbornness in one's beliefs, an irrational insensitivity to counterevidence, is a different kind of robustness...those who know *p* often lack a stubborn belief in *p*' (p.63). Williamson (2000, pp.7–8, 62–63, 86–87) takes a further step, linking the robustness of knowledge with persistence in the carrying through of actions. 'Action typically involves complex interaction with the environment; one needs continual feedback to bring it to a successful conclusion...Attributions of knowledge often explain the success of these interactions better than do the corresponding attributions of belief, even true belief' (p.8). Thus, whenever Bob *knows* that a certain puzzle can be solved, he will devote whatever time it takes to solve it, but not so when Bob (merely) *believes* that some puzzle has a solution.[12]

---

[12] Jim Joyce (personal communication, 2007) points out a problem with Williamson's view here. Joyce grants that knowing will produce persistence in action over and above believing—except in the following type of important case: Since both the mental state of believing and that of knowing are not transparent, Joyce asks what happens when some agent has an internal mental state consistent with knowing, but actually is wrong? One must conclude that the agent's actions would be just as persistent. However, since knowing is a factive mental state, regulated externally and therefore never false, one must also conclude that this type of persistence of action is due to what has turned out to be a false belief (albeit one experienced as knowledge). This argument is sound, but leads to a new problem, namely, the *post hoc* classifying of all mental states of failed knowledge as false belief. But how *is* one to classify them? Indeed, granting Williamson's externalist criterion—that knowing requires truth—such mental states clearly cannot be knowledge.

Here is my proposed solution. Although admittedly it is not desirable to add entities to epistemic ontology, because neither 'false belief' nor 'knowledge' satisfactorily specifies these state types, I propose that a separate mental state for 'knowing-that-turns-out-wrong' be considered. Animal actions argue in favor of such a proposal. Animals have mental states in which they have knowledge and they act upon these mental states. They are also wrong sometimes and, *pace* Joyce, they act in these cases with just as much vigor and perseverance. However, does one want to claim that these animals had false beliefs? No, since this would necessarily imply that they have the sophistication necessary for having beliefs generally—beliefs that are not all or none, but inherently graded. (For more on animals, see the subsection on 'non-human animals' in the later section, 'First-order and second-order knowledge and belief; believing what one knows; knowledge without (any sort of) belief.')

Various types of knowledge

Another important distinction between knowledge and belief is that knowledge, but not belief, comes in different kinds.[13] Aside from the most frequently dealt with *knowing that Z*, there is *knowing-how*, in the sense of having an ability, *knowing Y*, in the sense of being familiar with Y, and *knowing X from Y*, in the sense of being capable of making a discrimination.

Gilbert Ryle (1949, pp.28, 59–60) made, what has become the classic distinction between *knowing that* and *knowing-how*. Knowing that Z pertains to one knowing that Z is the case, while knowing-how to R, means that one has the ability to R. So, e.g., Ann *knows that* the answer to a particular problem involving solving certain types of equations is 4.00076. She knows because she looked it up in the index. However, she looked it up in the index because she does not yet have the *know-how* to solve that sort of problem. Cindy, on the other hand does have the know-how to solve that sort of problem, but when she arrives at her answer, she is not ready to say that she knows it to be the case, as she realizes that she might have made an error in one of the many steps in carrying it out.

There have been attempts to demonstrate that all knowing-that actually reduces to knowing-how. John Hartland-Swann, e.g., (1958, esp. p.58),[14] argues that every knowing that X can be construed as an ability or a knowing-how to answer a particular question to which X is the answer. Conversely, there have been arguments that knowing-how is a subspecies of knowing-that. For example, Jason Stanley and Timothy Williamson (2001) hold that knowing-how—while neither fully defined by nor reducible to terms applicable generally to knowing-that (pp.433–434)—is essentially involved with knowing 'ways of engaging in actions' (p.431). And for Stanley and Williamson, to know a *way* is a form of knowing that is 'no less propositional' than other examples of knowing-that (p.431); indeed for them '…to say someone knows how to *F* is always to ascribe to them knowledge-that' (p.426).

---

[13] Now it may be argued that belief also comes in different types. There are beliefs about facts like: 'I believe that our dog is barking.' And then there are beliefs like: 'Z believes in God,' and 'Q believes you should always arrive at least 10 minutes late for a dinner party.' I have argued (Brakel 2001) that these sorts of cultural and religious beliefs, as well as certain fixed phantasies of neurotic patients experienced and treated as beliefs, 'neurotic-beliefs' (e.g., a good-looking man who is convinced he is ugly), are not in fact beliefs-proper. These sorts of cognitive attitudes seem not to come in degrees, are often evidence insensitive, and in the extreme admit of no evidence—e.g., in the God case, what would count as evidence against God's existence for a believer? In short, since these 'beliefs' are not evidence regulated and do not aim at the truth (the definition of belief operative here), they cannot be beliefs-proper. (See also footnote 4.)

[14] See also Chisholm (1957, p.15) for more references to such arguments.

Other philosophers have extended the know-that/know-how distinction in interesting ways. David Lewis (1983, 1990), for instance, asks what sort of knowledge is needed to *know what it is like*. He answers (1983), regarding the taste of Vegemite, 'knowing what it is like is not the possession of information at all…Rather knowing what it is like is the possession of abilities: abilities to recognize, abilities to imagine, abilities to predict one's behavior by means of imaginative experiments' (p.131). He concludes (1990), '…knowing what an experience is like…is not knowing-that. It's knowing how' (p.516). David Armstrong (1973, p.177) finds that know-how is the sort of knowledge needed both for the capacity to discriminate X from Y, and for the ability to be acquainted or familiar with Z, where Z in Armstrong's example is someone, or some thing, about which one could have mental content. E.J. Lemmon (1967), while agreeing that there is a distinction to be made among different types of knowledge, contends that knowing-how and knowing-that are actually closer than either is to *knowing how to*. Using the example of driving a car, Lemmon explains that someone can know how it is done without knowing how to do it, concluding that the main difference is between '*practical* and *theoretical* information' (p.59).

Knowing X, in the sense of being familiar enough with X to be able to make a discrimination between X and Y, leads to a consideration of perceptual knowledge. Here the work of Alvin Goldman figures prominently. Speaking of his own goals, Goldman (1976) says:

> I am trying to fashion an account of knowing that focuses on more primitive and pervasive aspects of cognitive life, in connection with which…the term 'know' gets its application. A fundamental facet of animate life, both human and infra--human, is telling things apart, distinguishing predator from prey, for example, or a protective habitat from a threatening one. The concept of knowledge has its roots in this kind of cognitive activity. (p.791)

A reliablist,[15] for Goldman, knowledge (perceptual knowledge, but pointing the way toward knowledge in general) involves discrimination such that one must not only be able to differentiate between incompatible, but relevantly alternative, states of affairs, but to do so non-accidentally through appropriate causal connections such that knowledge of X is *reliably* produced when X is present, and knowledge of X *reliably* denied when X is not present. (pp.771–772, 790). Although he does not reduce all types of knowledge to either knowing-that or knowing-how, Goldman implies that at least in some cases, by having the kind of *reliable* ability or know-how necessary to be familiar enough with X to discriminate it from Y, one is in effect also demonstrating knowing-that.

---

[15] Reliabilism is briefly explained just below.

In his words (1976), 'I suggest that a person is said to know that p just in case he *distinguishes* or *discriminates* the truth of p from relevant alternatives' (p.772).[16]

Similarities between knowledge (knowing) and belief (believing)

Knowledge and belief are mental states

A mental state is a state of mind of an agent. Mental states come in various forms. The ones under discussion here are called mental or psychological attitudes—attitudes toward contents—and mental attitudes also come in various forms. There are conative attitudes, such as desire, in which the content is *to be brought about*, and cognitive attitudes, such as belief, in which the content of the attitude is regarded as *having come about*. (See Velleman 2000, pp.9–10, 111–112.) When I desire d, a cool drink of water, I would like d, my having a cool drink to be made the case. The direction is from my psychological state to the world. When I believe w, that there is a water fountain 20 feet from here, it is the case (from my point of view) that w, a water fountain, exists 20 feet from here. Here the direction is from the world to my mental state. In addition, then there are also *factive* mental attitudes, of which knowing is the most basic[17] (Williamson 2000, p.21). Contents of factive mental states also have come about in the world-to-mind direction, but whereas I can believe p even if p is not true, I can know p only if p is true. There is a tricky aspect to this. For belief, although I can believe p even if p is not true, I cannot believe p if I find out that p is not true. For knowledge, I can never be in the mental state of knowing p if p is not true—even if I am not in possession of the relevant facts. I can think I know p at time t (before I have learned the facts); but if p is not true, I was mistaken at time t, no matter when or if I learn the facts. If at time $t + 1$ I learn the facts and now know I was mistaken, I can correctly assert that at time t I thought I knew p, but that I was wrong.

---

[16] For Goldman (correctly in my view) the discriminator need have no concept of 'truth.' One can observe behavioral manifestations in which it is clear that an animal can reliably pick out that p (predator) is present, when p is present, and that q (prey) is not, when q is not. It is these behaviors, not the possession of a concept of truth, that constitute (as well as demonstrate) the 'truth' of p, and the not-'truth' of q for that animal.

[17] Others include perceiving and remembering.

Internalist accounts do not suffice for knowledge or belief

Not all philosophers agree that knowledge is a mental state.[18] Part of the difficulty comes from the notion that, with regard to the internal psychological aspect of both belief (true and false belief) and knowledge, both are identical, whereas the truth aspect necessary for knowledge comes externally, from the world. In this view, knowing is a mixture of mental and non-mental parts and therefore not a true mental state. Williamson (2000, pp.55–56) discusses the problem thus: 'The idea that the mental (or psychological) component of knowing is simply believing seems to be expressed in a remark by Stephen Stich, endorsed by Jaegwon Kim: "what knowledge adds to belief is psychologically irrelevant" (Stich 1978, p.574 quoted in Kim 1993, p.188)....' To the contrary, in the view held here (following Williamson), knowledge is a distinct mental state—not a conjunctive amalgam of belief plus something else. That is: 'To know is not merely to believe while various other conditions are met; it is to be in a new kind of state, a factive one...[which implies] the rejection of a conjunctive account of knowing' (Williamson 2000, pp.47–48).

The challenge conjunctive accounts of knowing present to the view of knowing as a singular factive mental state will be taken up later. (See the subsection 'The case for belief entailing knowledge' in the section on 'The priority of knowledge,' and footnote 42.) However, for now it is of interest, and counts as a point of similarity between knowledge and belief, to hold (as I do) that a strictly internalist account will not suffice for knowledge or belief. The case is straightforward with knowledge. As discussed above, the mental state of knowing 'p is q' when p *is* q, cannot be identical to the mental state of ~knowing 'p is q' when p *is not* q. Knowing as an attitude is partly determined by truth conditions in the world external to the subject. On the other hand, a belief that 'p is q' when p *is* q can seem identical to a belief that 'p is q,' when p *is not* q. The content of the true belief and that of the false belief can appear to be the same. Nonetheless, many hold that the content of beliefs cannot be fully determined internally, anymore than can the contents comprising attitudes of knowledge. This is readily demonstrated with the famous twin-earth cases (Hilary Putnam 1975), in which some earthling's belief about water—water is wet—is not the same as his/her twin earth doppleganger's belief—twin earth-water (t-water) is wet—no matter how identical the content seems and even if the neuronal firing patterns are identical. The earthling's belief is about *water*, while the twin-earthling's belief is about *t-water*, and since they are not having

---

[18] See, e.g., Hintikka 1962, esp p.82.

beliefs about the same content, the beliefs are different.[19] Thus, on this view, internalism is insufficient both for knowledge and belief—'If the content of a mental state can depend on the external world [in the belief case], so can the attitude to that content. Knowledge is such an attitude' (Williamson 2000, p.6).[20]

The proper causal chain

As was discussed above (see footnote 2), both knowledge and justified true belief must arrive at their content in appropriate ways to count as instances of knowledge or justified true belief. So, e.g., suppose I had a dream that my favorite uncle would call me in exactly 1 week. Then, exactly 1 week later, owing to the dream, when I heard the phone ring I had the belief that it was my favorite uncle. Now suppose further that it was in fact my uncle on the phone. Concerning his calling, I would have had a true, but unjustified, belief. Hallucinations that happen to contain content that is accurate—veridical hallucinations (see Armstrong 1973, p.171)—can be understood in the same way. The hallucinator hears a voice saying 'Come here now' and believes that there is an external person saying 'Come here now.' If on some occasion there *is* a person telling the hallucinator, 'Come here now,' the hallucinator's belief in this case will be true but unjustified to the extent that it is still is predicated on the hallucinatory, rather than the external voice.

Knowledge too must be obtained with the right 'pedigree.' Some years ago, I was running an experiment in which stimuli were presented subliminally, at the objective threshold for vision. This means that participants' conscious visual experience of the presented stimuli was nil. One task that participants were asked to perform was to indicate whether on a particular trial they thought a stimulus item or a blank was being presented, this after being informed that in this portion of the experiment they would receive blanks half the time and

---

[19] If an earthling is on twin earth and thinks 'I know this water is wet,' pointing to some body of *t-water*, this does not constitute knowledge, but an unjustified true belief. The earthling is right but for the wrong reasons. He/she has taken the *t-water* sample, which happens to be wet, as *water*.

[20] This is not to deny that internalism about beliefs is different from internalism about knowledge. Internalism about beliefs leads to problems individuating differing contents; but the different beliefs with different contents are still all beliefs, and a strict internalist account would still get that right. Strict internalism about knowledge, on the other hand, would have more profound consequences. External truth values contribute to the determination of whether a mental state is one of knowing at all; there is no mental state consisting in 'false knowing'; knowledge that is false is incoherent. However, see footnote 12.

stimulus items half the time, and that they should try to respond with that information in mind. Most participants dutifully attended to the stimuli and 'guessed,' with half of their responses 'blank' and half 'stimulus item.' One subject refused to participate (although he only told the experimenter this after the fact). He did not really pay any attention to the stimuli, but said 'blank' on every trial. Later, he revealed his reasoning: 'Since I never saw any-thing, anyway, I "know" that actually they were all blanks no matter what you said.' He was right exactly 50% of the time—but he had no knowledge—neither on those trials on which he happened to be correct nor on those about which he was wrong.[21]

Anti-luminosity: Belief and knowledge are not transparent mental states

A luminous condition is defined as one in which, whenever it obtains in an agent, the agent knows that it obtains. The conditions of being in pain and having things appear to us in whatever ways they do are examples used to dem-onstrate conditions considered luminous, transparent, and directly accessible first personally to the agent in question (Williamson 2000, pp.95–96). The case for anti-luminosity with regard to both knowledge and belief is perhaps most simply stated thus: We can believe things and we can know things without believing, knowing, or being aware that we believe or know them. We have no privileged access; not to the proper typing of the mental states we are in, nor to the content of these mental states. Taking a strong anti-luminosity position, Williamson (2000), without denying that there is much that we can know, calls us 'cognitively homeless' (p.94), claiming that there is no central core of trans-parent mental states about which we cannot go wrong. (pp.93–113).[22]

The position that knowing is non-luminous seems most obviously true about performances, i.e., knowings-how, as, e.g., A.D. Woozley (1953) states, '[Take] A claiming that he doesn't know how to do something, and B replying

---

[21] Accounts of knowing the contents of subliminally presented items will be given, at length, in the next major section.

[22] Williamson's (2000, pp.96–98) claim is more extreme than the position I take. For him, even feeling cold or pain at a particular time and situations like 'X appears to him as X.' do not count as luminous. He does not offer the usual arguments that someone might not have the concepts 'cold' or 'knowing.' Instead, Williamson advances a sorites paradox type of argument that involves a continuum where what constitutes cold cannot accu-rately be determined as time and temperature changes occur incrementally. (See Chapter 3 for much more on the sorites paradox and sorites paradox arguments.) For the pur-poses of this chapter however, there is no disagreement that both belief and knowledge are non-luminous mental states about which we have no privileged access.

that he (A) knows perfectly well how to do it…B can often follow up …by showing A that he (A) does know' (p.152). (See also Ryle 1949, p.53.) However, Woozley himself adds that this is no less true for knowings-that: 'knowing is not self-certifying, as you can know but not know that you know, just as much as you can wrongly think you know and not know that you're wrongly think-ing it' (p.172). Along these same lines, Armstrong (1973) explains that, 'it is logically possible to be mistaken about, or unaware of the existence of, any of our current mental states just as much as any other state of affair in the world' (p.146). Moreover, 'It is possible…for A to know that *p* and *disbelieve* he knows it' (p.212 [my emphasis]). (See also Danto1968, p.153 and Margolis 1973, p.15 who also hold this view.)

As for mis-typing one sort of mental state for another, this everyday occur-rence stands out even more clearly when working with psychoanalytic patients. (See Brakel 2001, 2009, esp Chapters 7 and 8.) Conative attitudes (mental states), such as desires and wishes, not only color beliefs, but can also be mis-taken for beliefs. The trope of the parched desert traveler's oasis mirage is made real by patients who, e.g., are so hungry for love from indifferent per-sons, that they take neutral (or even frankly negative) facts as positive indica-tors. Thus spouse A, desiring love from spouse B, interprets B's phone call telling him that she will have to cancel their plans as a sign that she really loves him. A says to his analyst, 'Yes, she cancelled, but she called first, she really cares.' This suggests that he experiences his desire for her to love him as a belief that she does.

Patients in analysis even more frequently confuse distinct cognitive mental states, one for another. For example, certain phantasies—attitudes with content that one phantasizes or imagines to be the case—are often regarded, experienced, and, in important ways, serve to function as beliefs. However, clearly, they are not beliefs; they are not regulated by evidence and do not aim at the truth. Take, for instance, a patient who, despite his own ample evidence to the contrary, fixedly believes that no one likes him and, in many ways, acts as though it is the case that nobody does. I have termed these fixed phantasy-laden mental states 'neurotic-beliefs' (Brakel 2001, 2009), maintaining that in part the most troubling, life-disturbing, pathological nature of neurosis is caused by this very mis-categorizing; e.g., when these phantasy-like neurotic-beliefs are mistaken for beliefs-proper and thereby used to guide (really mis-guide) the patient's real-world actions (2001, p.384).

Other patients make an even more serious categorizing mistake, confound-ing phantasies with knowledge. There are, for instance, patients who engage in physically self-mutilating behaviors such as cutting themselves. These are most often very complex patients, and yet one common 'reason' for their physically self-destructive behavior often emerges: Cutters cut because they 'know' that this is the only way that they can feel better. That this sort of mis-typing (mistaking phantasies for knowledge) often contributes to more severe psychopathology derives from one of the important differences between beliefs and knowledge discussed above, namely, that knowledge, more so than belief, resists change and leads to persistence in acting in accord with its content.

For our current purpose, what follows is perhaps the most important implication of knowing as a non-transparent, non-luminous mental state about which we have no privileged access, either in terms of content or mental state attitude type: If there is no luminosity there can be no necessity that knowing p entails knowing that you know p or even believing that you know p. Three vital questions follow: 1) What is the nature of the relation of first-order knowledge (knowing p) to second-order knowledge and second-order belief (i.e., knowing or believing that you know p, expressed as KK and BK, respectively)?[23] 2) Must one believe what one knows (BK)? and 3) Can one have knowledge without any belief at all, i.e., with neither subsequent nor prior belief? In other words, must knowledge entail belief (K→B)? These matters are so fundamental that they warrant a section of their own, which follows forthwith.

First- and second-order knowledge and belief; believing what one knows; knowledge without (any sort of) belief

Background

Chisholm (1957) warns that even if there is a sense that knowing does entail believing: '…we must not think of knowing as being, in any sense, a "species" of believing…The relation of knowing to believing…is not that of a falcon to bird or airedale to dog[24]; it is more like that of arriving to traveling. *Arriving* entails *traveling*—a man cannot arrive unless he has traveled—but arriving is not a species of traveling' [his emphasis] (pp.17–18). Merrill Ring (1977) argues that Chisholm cannot have both that 1) knowing entails believing and 2) knowing is not a species of believing. Ring explains that Chisholm wants to 'save' the thesis that knowledge entails belief, but that the example of traveling and arriving 'is so far from upholding his view that it belongs to mine' (p.59). Ring's view uses the very same example to demonstrate that knowledge cannot

---

[23] K stands for knowing; B for believing. What can be known or believed includes both content and mental state type.

[24] Chisholm (1957, p.18) attributes these examples of dis-analogy to Ryle.

entail belief: 'Arriving does not entail traveling—it entails *having* traveled [Ring's emphasis]. When one has arrived, one is no longer traveling. Similarly, when one does come to know what was previously believed, the believing like the traveling is over' (p.59). Ring (1977) goes on to describe that in knowing something the knower cannot be trying to find out what is already known, as distinct from believing something in which the believer will be trying to find out what is merely believed (p.59).

However, Ring's position, although an emphatic denial that knowledge entails belief, is an equally strong avowal that knowing entails *having believed*. Obviously, looked at from the account I am trying to advance here, this temporal entailment is no improvement. So, here, for instance, is some evidence against Ring's view. In the negative hallucination case presented above, Dr. N had no prior beliefs regarding the content that he both knew but did not know he knew. Further, prior to his state of knowledge he made no attempts to gain the knowledge; in fact he tried to not-know it. On the other hand, take a case of someone knowing the answer to something but not being able to bring it to mind. The agent in this situation knows that he/she knows. Yet the content of the knowledge remains unconscious. The agent tries hard to bring the answer to consciousness, but experiences difficulty in retrieving the unconsciously known content. Again, no prior beliefs are involved

Others, despite having views largely similar to Ring's, agree with me (to an extent) regarding the problem with knowing *necessarily* entailing having believed. For example, Pritchard's (1950) account first makes a claim identical to Ring's that knowing, as a mental state, entails 'not-believing,' in the very particular sense of not currently believing. He then argues that because knowledge and belief are both irreducible mental states, knowledge can neither be a species of belief, nor entail ongoing belief, even though '...believing is a stage we *sometimes* [my emphasis] reach in the endeavour to attain knowledge' (p.88).[25]

Still, Pritchard's account is problematic in another way. He holds that the very separateness of knowledge from belief is predicated on complete transparency or luminosity of each of these mental states: '...whenever we know something, we do, or at least can, by reflecting directly know that we are knowing it, and that whenever we believe something, we similarly do or can directly know that we are believing it and not knowing it' (p.86). Transparency, just

---

[25] Philosophers such as Ring and Pritchard endorse the 'historical' position (i.e., knowing following after believing), a position that according to Williamson (2000, pp.41–42) stands in sharp contrast to those embracing the 'standard analysis' on which knowing entails ongoing believing.

like luminosity, of course amounts to knowing that you know and knowing that you believe; epistemic capacities that are far from established.

Clearly then, the position I take in this chapter is far different from those of Chisholm and Pritchard and Ring, and it includes the following: 1) Knowing and believing are each separate mental states. 2) Knowing and believing are not luminous or transparent, meaning there is no privileged access. Thus neither KK (knowing that and what you know) and KB (knowing that and what you believe) nor BK (believing what you know) obtains routinely. 3) Knowing does not imply ongoing or prior believing, not conceptually and not temporally. Can this view hold up? In the words of the title of this section, can a case be made for:

1) First-order knowledge without second-order knowledge (K but not necessarily KK);
2) Knowing without second-order believing what you know (K but not necessarily BK); and finally
3) Knowledge, without knowledge entailing belief of any sort, including prior belief (K, but not K→ B)?

The following subsections present examples that argue for one or more of the above claims. (Negative hallucinations warrant such a subsection, but are not included here as they were described at length earlier in the chapter.)

Savant syndrome

As reported in Wikipedia (consulted on 9 March 2007), Savant Syndrome (this term replacing 'idiot savant') represents a disorder marked by any one of a group of unusual cognitive abilities, usually associated with autism or related disturbances. The e-reference states:

> Savant Syndrome ... can also be acquired in an accident or illness, typically one that injures or impairs the left side of the brain. There is some research that suggests that it can be induced, which might support the view that savant abilities are latent within all people but are obscured by the normal functioning intellect... Most autistic savants have very extensive mental abilities, called *splinter skills*. They can memorize facts, numbers, license plates, maps, and extensive lists of sports and weather statistics. Some savants can mentally note and then recall perfectly a very long sequence of music, numbers, or speech. Some, dubbed mental calculators, can do exceptionally fast arithmetic, including prime factorization. Other skills include precisely estimating distances and angles by sight, calculating the day of the week for any given date over the span of tens of thousands of years, and being able to accurately gauge the passing of time without a clock. Usually these skills are concrete, non-symbolic, right hemisphere skills, rather than left hemisphere skills, which tend to be more sequential, logical, and symbolic.[26]

---

[26] Wikipedia cites Darold Treffert, M.D., Clinical Professor of Psychiatry, University of Wisconsin, as the reference for this material.

When persons with savant syndrome are asked to perform any of their splinter skills—say picking out the day of the week for several dates in different years across thousands of years—assuming that the savants get the answers right, they clearly know the answers. That this ability involves first-order knowledge is clear. However, what else does such a splinter skill entail? Certainly there seem to be no beliefs necessary to arrive at these answers—the savants know the right answers without any prior beliefs about which days of the week fall on particular dates. Further, when savants demonstrate their skill for the first time, as far as experimenters and observers can tell, these savants have neither secondary knowledge nor even secondary belief as to whether or not they can perform this task. Likely after many flawless performances, a secondary belief in their own ability to know grows; but this is conceptually trivial.

A (fictional) French Canadian who claims to know no English history

Colin Radford (1966, pp.2–7) introduces Jean, a fictional French Canadian who claims to know no English history. After all, Jean explains, this is not what is taught at French-Canadian schools. Nonetheless, he gets involved in trying to answer questions on this subject for cash, and he misses a few. Then he is asked when Queen Elizabeth died. He responds, 'Ohh…Mmm…Sixteen-oh-three?' To which his questioner replies, 'Yes! Now tell me you haven't done any history!…(sarcastically): That was just a guess, was it?' (p.2). Jean then proceeds to answer when Elizabeth's successor, James the First, died, 'Oh… Ah…James the First. So he's sixteen-oh-three to…to…sixteen twenty-five?' (p.3). Now the questioner, affirming that Jean's answer is correct, is more emphatic that Jean must have learned these English history dates. Jean says, 'Well, I certainly don't remember. As far as I can tell I'm just guessing' (p.3). Finally, after getting a few more questions right about Tudor and Stuart royalty, Jean himself is impressed by the detail of his own correct responses, and realizes that he must have learned these things. He then comes up with the occasion—it was as a punishment that the dates of particular kings and queens had to be memorized. However, Jean comments that he had completely forgotten, and his questioner believes him, 'Freudian forgetting, I expect' (p.3).

Radford (1966) analyzes the case as one in which Jean knows P (the dates he got right), but 'was not certain, or sure, or confident that P. Indeed he was fairly certain that his answer…was wrong, *i.e.*, that not-P, since he believed it to be a pure guess' (p.4). Radford continues that if the case of Jean 'is a possible one…it shows that a man may know that P even though he is *neither* sure that P, and indeed is fairly sure that not-P, *nor* justified in being sure, *etc.*, that P!' (p.4). Further Jean did not know that he knew until the questioner told him that his answers were correct. For Radford this means 'Jean knows at the first level—even though he is not sure…and that these considerations do not exist or operate at the second level' (p.6). In other words, 'he is not aware, does not realize, i.e., he does not know, that he knows any [English] history' (p.7).

Jean, like people with savant syndrome, can have 1) knowledge without belief prior to or about that knowledge, and 2) first-order knowledge without second-order knowledge or belief. Further, not only is it possible for Jean to know P without believing P, he can in fact believe not-P.

The chicken-sexer and horserace picker

Goldman (1975, pp.114–116) presents the case of a professional chicken-sexer who, despite having the know-how to distinguish between male and female chicks with remarkable accuracy, has no idea how he does it. A similar case, that of Jones the picker of horserace winners, is offered by D. S. Mannison (1976, pp.142–147). Jones too has predictive know-how; he can choose the winning horse with great consistency, but like the chicken-sexer, he is mystified by his own technique. Both men clearly have know-how and, regarding each of many individual situations, they show that they know-that too. The chicken-sexer knows, for instance, that Chick X is female, Chick Y is male, and Jones knows that Fleetfoot will win Race 1, Firefly Race 2, etc. However, do they have second-order knowledge? Can Jones know that he will know the outcome of an upcoming race?

The answer for Mannison (1976) turns on Jones' experience. If it is 1950 and Jones has just started the winning racehorse-picking business, he cannot know that he will know, even though he indeed does know that Sure Thing will be the winner. However, if it is 1974 and he has been selecting the winning horses for every race for more than two decades, he can know that he will pick the winner of a specific upcoming race. Further for Mannison (1976), Jones would be justified in claiming to know solely on the grounds that he always does pick the winner of a race. This second-order knowledge is based on knowing of one's know-how or *knowing that I can and shall* (p.144), and it is not the same as know-how. Wittgenstein (1953) in *Philosophical Investigations* (section #324) advances the same position: '…I am as certain that I shall be able to continue the series, as I am that this book will drop to the ground when I let it go; and that I should be no less astonished if I suddenly and for no obvious reason got stuck…than I should if the book remained hanging in the air… What could justify the certainty *better* than success?' (p.106).

However, let us return to Jones in 1950. Here Mannison (1976) describes him as having neither second-order knowledge nor second-order belief about his knowing that a particular horse, No.4, will win, while in fact disbelieving what he knows. Speaking for Jones, Mannison (1976) writes, "'As there are twelve horses in the race, and I have no horseracing expertise, I have no reason to believe that No. 4 will win…the odds against No. 4 winning are eleven to one. As these are formidable odds, I would only be reasonable in holding that some horse other than No. 4 will win'" (p.147). So the case of Jones, similar to that of Jean, also demonstrates that one can have knowledge of P without second-order knowledge or belief of P, and in fact with belief of not-P.

What about second-order knowledge and belief and the chicken-sexer? In the natural course of events, it would appear that the chicken-sexer, once he became established, would form beliefs that the chicks he 'knew' to be males really were males and those he 'knew' to be females really were females. These beliefs and their justification, like those of Jones and his horserace predictions, clearly would be entirely predicated on the success of his chicken-sexing know-how and the many resultant instances of his demonstrating that he knows-that.

However, Goldman (1975, p.115) sets up an interesting case: Suppose the chicken-sexer is persuaded that his performances of late have been bad. Assuming his abilities are intact, he would still be correctly sexing chicks, i.e., still possessing his know-how, so that the resultant instances of chick-sexing (knowings-that) would still be correct. The chicken-sexer, under these conditions, would still have first-order knowledge. However, now he would be without any true and justified second-order beliefs a) about his know-how, b) about the individual cases, and c) about the *knowing that he can and shall*, described by Mannison. In fact he would have false beliefs about his outcomes.

Although Goldman (1975) appears to agree regarding the first-order knowledge, he introduces confusing belief-talk where it is most inappropriate:

> Why…do we credit knowledge to the chicken-sexer…? The answer…is given by the causal theory of knowing…there is a certain kind of causal connection between the fact that p and S's *belief* [my italics] that p…In the chicken-sexing case the fact that the chick is male causes S to *believe* [my italics] that it is male (p.116).

Actually his *belief* (second-order) about the sex of the chick can be distorted by what he is falsely told about his performances, but not his *knowledge* (first order) about its sex. Assuming he is still sexing the chicks correctly, he still *knows* that a male chick is male, even if he can no longer believe in his knowledge. Thus, emending Goldman's statement above, without contesting the causal theory of knowing, and in fact repeating most of his own words, I hold:

> Why…do we credit knowledge to the chicken–sexer…? The answer…is given by the causal theory of knowing…there is a certain kind of causal connection between the

fact that p and S's *knowing* that p. In the chicken-sexing case, the fact that the chick is male causes S to *know* it is male. In addition, let us add that this is the case no matter what he is told and subsequently falsely *believes* about the matter and/or if he has *no beliefs* about the matter whatsoever![27]

Thus whether the chicken-sexer has false second-order beliefs, predicated on the false information given him, or true second-order beliefs, predicated on his experience and memories of his remarkable record of successful instances of correct sexing of chicks, his first-order knowledge is intact and not reliant on beliefs of any sort.

The winning-racehorse picker and the chicken-sexer are examples of know-how leading to instances of first-order knowing-that, all requiring no prior (or concomitant) belief. Further, both cases demonstrate that such first-order knowledge can exist without second-order true belief or second order knowledge about what is known, and indeed with false belief about what is known.

The duck/rabbit dual figure and dream drawing

The duck/rabbit dual figure (see Figure 2.1) and other such ambiguous figures have been used in many psychological experiments. Although the psychologists did not set out to explore first- and second-order knowledge, there is one group of experiments that bears on this matter. Following earlier work,[28] David Chambers and Daniel Reisberg (1985) presented the duck/rabbit stimulus figure to subjects who were unfamiliar with it. After the subjects had had enough time to form a mental image, the figure was removed. Subjects were asked what they had seen. All of the subjects who reported both a duck and a rabbit were excused from the rest of the study. The remaining subjects were asked to consider the other ambiguous stimulus figures they had worked with in practice sessions and then to internally re-examine their mental image of the figure (the duck/rabbit) they had been presented. Despite this, they reported only the single original animal—duck or rabbit. Next, they were given hints about the missing answer, and again asked to review their mental image. Again, most gave just the unitary response. Finally the subjects were asked to draw

---

[27] One might wonder about prior beliefs contributing to the successes of the chicken-sexer; in other words, do prior beliefs contribute to his knowledge? However, Goldman (1975) has taken pains to specify that the chicken-sexer 'is ignorant of *how* he tells the sex of the chick' (p.114), i.e., has no idea of his technique. This implies that he does not have a set of consistent beliefs leading him to his ultimate conclusion; so we have instead another case of knowledge without belief.

[28] See also Reed and Johnsen 1975.

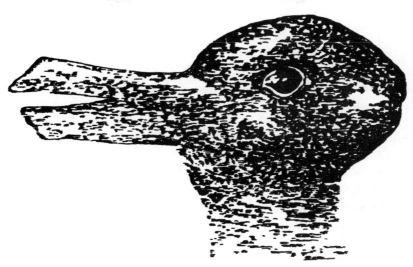

Fig. 2.1 The duck/rabbit.

their mental image. Now, in looking at their drawings both duck and rabbit emerged for all of the subjects.

The question bearing on first- and second-order knowledge concerns the status of the duck or rabbit figure that could not be recognized until the subjects drew the mental image of the presented stimulus figure. Take Subject A who immediately reported that in her mental image she saw a duck, but nothing else; she saw no rabbit—not until the very last step in the experiment, when she was asked to draw her mental image of the figure originally presented. At this point, and with some surprise, she looked at her own drawing and saw not just a duck, but also a rabbit. What can be made of this? It is uncontestable that throughout the process, Subject A had both first- and second-order knowledge of the duck. She not only knew that a duck was presented, she knew that she knew. However, the more interesting matter is: What did she know about the rabbit and when? For most of the experiment, it *seemed* that she had no knowledge about the rabbit. However, when she was asked to draw her own mental image, *presto*, a rabbit emerged. Once she recognized the rabbit she had second-order knowledge of it. I maintain that *all along* she had first-order knowledge of the rabbit, but that this first-order knowledge was unconscious. This is strikingly similar to the negative hallucination case presented at length in the beginning of the chapter. Dr N had unconscious first-order knowledge of my having fallen asleep. Only after reporting his thinly disguised dream did he have conscious second-order knowledge; and he never recaptured his first-order experience of knowing that I had fallen asleep. Subject A, after she drew her mental image, could see and know both duck and rabbit, at which point she had both first- and second-order knowledge of both of the figures.

Consistent with these experimental findings are some examples from clinical psychoanalytic work. Although these data are of necessity more complex than those from psychology experiments, it has been found that certain patients in analysis, when asked to draw particular elements from their dreams, can sometimes discover (un-cover) something they had known but not wanted to know. (See Fisher 1957; Slap 1976; and Brakel 1993.) In other words patients can, after viewing their drawing of a dream element, arrive at first- and second-order knowledge of something that had been repressed and therefore known only in an unconscious first-order way. This resembles closely the situation just described in the duck/rabbit drawing experiment. For example, consider my patient Ms. P.[29] She remembered that her father had been physically abusive to her mother and her brothers. She remembered that he killed two family pets. However, after 3 years in analysis she was struggling with whether or not she had been physically abused or perhaps sexually molested by her father or someone else. Ms. P reported the following dream: 'It is a life-and-death situation. Either kill or be killed. I'd never shot anyone before, but I shot this guy. I had a weird gun with itty-bitty tear drop bullets.' She associated to several elements, but said nothing about the gun. When I pointed this out to her, she said: 'It was a weird gun, lots of bullets, like a machine gun, but it didn't look like that, more square, like a hand-held fertilizer or a sifter with a handle; squeeze it and shoot all the bullets. I can't describe the gun.' At this point I asked Ms. N to draw the gun. (see Figure 2.2). As soon as the drawing was complete she said, 'Now the handle looks like a big limp penis. And the teardrop bullets something reproductive—sperm. But I don't want it to be; I'd rather bury it. I think something really did happen and I say I want to remember but I really don't [want to].'

Note that I am not suggesting that Ms. N, on the basis of this dream, could now *know* whether or not she was abused. My clinical epistemological claims are far more modest. All I am saying is that when Ms. N dreamt of guns and associated to handheld fertilizers, she had penises and sperm on her mind. She knew in a first-order and unconscious way of her worries about the aggressive and sexual misuse of penises and sperm. Penises and sperm were then

---

[29] This material is taken from Brakel 1993, pp.363–64.

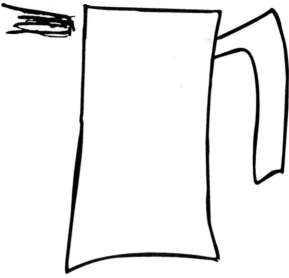

Fig. 2.2 Ms. N's drawing of dream element.[30]

disguised through the dream work[31] to guns and bullets, and then in her associations to sifters and fertilizers. Although both guns and fertilizers were rather thin disguises, it took the drawing of the dream element for Ms. N to know about her unconscious first-order knowledge in a second-order and conscious form.

Before the subjects and patients were asked to draw their mental or dream images, they had both first- and second-order knowledge of some things—e.g., the duck, and the gun in the dream. However, they had only first-order unconscious knowledge of some other things—the rabbit and the penis and sperm. Note that this first-order unconscious knowledge was unaccompanied by beliefs of any sort, and, as is true for all knowledge that is first order only, no knowledge of what they knew. When we add that this knowledge was not only just first order, but also unconscious, we add that the subjects and patients did

---

[30] The original version of this figure was published in the *Journal of the American Psychoanalytic Association*. Used with permission © 1993 American Psychoanalytic Association. All rights reserved.

[31] More on the nature of dreams can be found in Chapters 3 and 4 of this volume, and specifically on the dream work in Chapter 4. (See also Brakel 2009, Chapter 4.) Of course, for the original account, see Freud 1900.

not even know that they knew. They had no awareness that there was anything to know beyond the duck, and beyond the gun.[32]

Subliminal experiments

The examples in this section should make it even clearer that one can have first-order knowledge without any sort of belief—no prior belief, and no second-order belief—and no second-order knowledge about what is known. In subliminal experiments, subjects are presented stimulus items in such a way that they can have no conscious awareness of what has been presented. In some circumstances, namely under conditions that are at the objective threshold for detection, not only are subjects not aware of *what* item has been presented, they cannot even determine *that* an item has been presented. Despite this, such experiments demonstrate that subjects can gain what can best be considered first-order knowledge even under these stringent conditions.

For a first example take a well-known phenomenon in psychology called the mere exposure effect. In a classic experiment, William Kunst-Wilson and Robert Zajonc (1980) presented subjects a series of irregular polygons subliminally under subjective threshold conditions. (This means that subjects had no subjective awareness of seeing the polygons.) Next, each of these polygons was presented supraliminally (in full conscious awareness) and paired with an irregular polygon that had not been presented before. For each pair, subjects were asked two questions: One question concerned which of the two polygons they recognized, and the other asked which of the two they liked better. The recognition results were at chance; subjects were not aware of seeing the polygons, so they did not recognize them. However, when subjects were asked which of the two polygons they liked better, the results were significantly in favor of the polygon that had been presented previously. Although the subjects did not know that they knew the polygons that had been presented to them, they knew them in the sense of discriminating them from those that had not been presented, by liking them better. The subjects had first-order unconscious knowledge, but no second-order knowledge of (nor beliefs about) the polygons they had been presented earlier.

In another experiment, this one done at the objective detection threshold, subjects were not even aware that a stimulus was presented, much less what it was. The subjects were all social phobics. Researchers (Shevrin, Bond, Brakel, Hertel, and Williams 1996) presented two sets of words to each subject—one set

---

[32] One might ask: Why not infer first-order unconscious beliefs as well as unconscious first-order knowledge? This question will be taken up at length later in the Section titled 'Unconscious knowledge/unconscious belief.'

representing the subject's unconscious conflict and another set representing the subject's conscious symptom.[33] Each subject had his/her own individualized sets of words. Both sets of unique words were presented to each subject both subliminally (at the objective threshold) and supraliminally (in full awareness). Evoked-response potentials (ERPs), which are electrical measures of brain wave activity, were recorded during the presentations. Using a mathematically sophisticated time–frequency information analysis, whereby certain features of the ERPs can be used to test how well the ERPs to a certain class of stimuli can themselves be classified, we found the following. Across subjects, the time–frequency features classified the ERPs to the subliminally presented unconscious conflict words significantly better than they did the ERPs to the subliminally presented conscious symptom words; whereas supraliminally the reverse was true—ERPs to the supraliminally presented conscious symptom words were classified by the time–frequency features significantly more successfully than the ERPs from the supraliminally presented unconscious conflict words. Later in the experiment, when subjects were given a list of all of the words presented and asked to put them in categories, the conscious symptom words were placed in a single category, while the unconscious conflict words were dispersed over three or more categories. Both sets of results suggest that words associated with the subjects' symptoms and words representing their unconscious conflicts were experienced quite differently. Unlike the case with their conscious symptom words, subjects did not have second-order conscious knowledge of the words representing their own unconscious conflicts. Despite this, their brain responses gave evidence of first-order unconscious knowledge in that when these words were presented outside of consciousness (subliminally), they cohered very well for the subject's brain, just as they had for the psychoanalytic clinicians.

---

[33] Two psychoanalytic clinicians interviewed each subject extensively while the text of the interviews was recorded. Psychological tests were also administered and recorded. The interviewers and two other psychoanalysts reviewed the data from the texts of the interviews and the tests and then selected words that they all agreed best represented the subject's unconscious conflict—in other words, the unconscious source of the subject's symptom. These words were unique and quite different for each subject. For example, the name of a subject's sibling could be one of the words, if that sibling was central in a subject's unconscious conflict. The clinicians also picked out the words from the interviews and tests that best represented each subject's conscious symptom. These words, while not uniform among the subjects, had much in common. For example, words capturing one's anxiety would be present in the conscious symptom word set of many of the subjects.

A final example comes from an experiment done with spider phobics. Howard Shevrin, Michael Snodgrass, James Abelson, Ramesh Kuswaha, and I (in preparation) presented spider-phobic subjects subliminal stimuli consisting of line drawings of spiders and drawings of rectangles. All the stimuli were delivered at the objective detection threshold, meaning that subjects had no conscious awareness when and even that stimuli were presented, much less of their contents. ERPs were collected during 80 presentations—40 of spiders and 40 of rectangles delivered in randomized orders. Prior to and following the presentations, subjects rated their fear of spiders on several dimensions on an instrument called a visual analog scale (VAS). The findings of interest for our purposes concern an early component of the ERP, called N100. A negative going (hence the 'N') wave-form in the ERP occurring 100 ms after the presentation of stimuli, the N100 is associated with attention. The bigger a spider phobic's N100 response was to the spider pictures compared to N100 responses to the rectangle pictures, the greater was his/her VAS improvement. This means that the more a spider-phobic's brain behavior indicated discrimination between the spider pictures and the rectangle pictures (and in this sense *knowing* spiders from rectangles), the more improved was the phobic response. However, all of this was entirely unconscious. No subject had any notion of whether a spider or rectangle stimulus had been presented on any trial. No subject had any notion that they were making this discrimination. Finally, subjects were not even aware that they were giving responses that indicated a lessening of their phobic symptom. In a later debriefing it was clear that they believed that their response to spiders was unchanged. No second-order knowledge was available, even though there was brain and behavioral evidence of first-order unconscious knowing (in the sense of discriminating) spider from rectangle stimuli. Subjects did not know that they knew, they did not believe what they knew, and no prior belief formed the foundation of their knowledge.[34]

Neurotic-beliefs

The phenomenon of neurotic-belief (which I have discussed at length elsewhere, see Brakel 2001, 2009, Chapter 7) demonstrates another way in which one can know without believing what one knows. Most neurotic persons (and patients) have central phantasies, which are treated as beliefs, and have some of beliefs' causal and functional roles—this despite the important fact that

---

[34] For an opposing view to the one offered here with respect to the last two experiments, see Jones (1971) who argues against 'Attributing knowledge...on the grounds of certain suppositions about ...brain states' (p.23).

unlike beliefs, neurotic beliefs do not aim at the truth and are not regulated by evidence. Take, for instance, Mr. R who was brutally beaten many times by his father as a child. Now a very successful business man, middle aged and homosexual, he behaves in ways seemingly designed to never attract any man, even as he longs for sex, marriage, and male companionship. Through work in analysis, Mr. R first came to see that his characteristic overly dramatic style alternating with cool indifference was not likely to attract any of the men he was interested in attracting. We then began to understand the purpose of these behaviors. Over the decades, he had developed a complex phantasy (partly unconscious and partly conscious but irrational) that worked to explain his past problems and prevent future ones. The phantasy as we constructed it looked like this: Mr. R neurotically-believed that his father's damaging acts had been largely caused by his own lively (and very normal) little boy activities directed toward his father. So he neurotically-believed that as long as he was the opposite of normal—either too histrionic or too cold—not only would this sort of thing never happen again, it would also undo the past. Now Mr. R was not a psychotic person; he was competent and sophisticated and functioned well in the world. Clearly he *knew* that his father's sadistic physically damaging behavior owed mostly to his father's serious psychopathology and moral turpitude. He *knew* that behaving either with outrageous flamboyance or with cold self-containment could not guarantee future safety. Further, of course, he *knew* that the present cannot effect the past. Despite this, his neurotic-belief interfered with his rational capacities to believe what he knew. Mr. R had knowledge without believing what he knew.[35]

Non-human animals

Several authors grapple with the notion of animal knowledge. Shope (1983) states: 'We may say of a dog that it knows which bag holds the meat or knows that there is meat in this bag, without thereby implying that the dog accepts propositions' (p.182, n.10). But Shope acknowledges that, for some authors, granting that animals have knowledge implies attributing beliefs to them. Armstrong (1973), in discussing animal knowledge, starts out directly claiming that if there is knowledge then there is belief: 'If A [an animal] perceives that something is the case...then it is entailed that A knows that that thing is the case. And "A knows that p" entails "A believes that p"...Now it seems obvious that the dog perceives that a cat is streaking across the lawn...So the dog acquires knowledge and, if he acquires knowledge, acquires beliefs' (p.27).

---

[35] Is there something similar, although highly rationally based and not psychopathological, in skeptics who systematically refuse to believe what they know?

However, later, Armstrong leaves room for another interpretation, one more congenial to the view taken in this chapter, that knowledge precedes belief: 'If things of the sort X act upon an animal's sense organs, and, as a result, the animal proves able to act in a discriminating way toward the object which acted upon it, differentiating it from something which is not X, the animal can be credited with at least a *simple* concept of X' (p.63).[36]

Goldman (1977, p.118) describes the behavior of ticks as 'believing' that a certain odor (butyric acid, a component of human sweat) and a certain temperature (37°C) are indicators of a good place to suck blood. He goes on to describe an appropriate, natural selection-based causal connection between these 'beliefs' of ticks and the fact that these conditions are good for sucking blood. Because there is this appropriate causal connection, Goldman states: 'The causal theory of knowing, therefore, would vindicate the claim that the tick not only has innate true belief, but that it has innate knowledge' (p.118). I am convinced about knowledge—beyond the know-how involved in sucking, ticks discriminate good targets from not good ones, knowing-that this one or that one is worth the energy investment. But why do beliefs have to be a prior part of this picture? On my view they do not; and Goldman once again (as above with regard to the chicken-sexer) talks of beliefs, instead of knowledge. Tick knowledge accounts for the phenomenon in question more elegantly. (See the next section on 'Unconscious knowledge/unconscious belief' for the argument supporting this claim against Goldman's move and others like it.)

Conclusions on first- and second-order knowledge and beliefs

These cases demonstrate several classes of counter-examples to KK and BK (second-order knowing and believing) and thereby to luminosity. They also show various disconnects between knowledge and belief (prior, concomitant, and subsequent belief). In fact in none of these examples does knowledge entail belief; rather we have many cases with knowledge but no belief. Savants, and Jean the French-Canadian English history 'student,' do not have any beliefs at all about what they know[37] at least until after the fact of the performance. Likewise, people with negative hallucinations have no beliefs about what they know until someone reveals the content of the negative hallucination to them. The chicken-sexer and winning-racehorse picker early in their careers

---

[36] Armstrong unfortunately (from my viewpoint) still stops short of equating having a concept with knowledge, and seems to leave open whether or not belief is entailed by this sort of discrimination as a function of concept possession.

[37] Jean actually believed he had no knowledge of English history.

might even disbelieve what they know. The duck/chicken subjects, until they have made their drawings, believe only half of what they know. Participants in the subliminal experiments never believe anything about the contents of the stimuli they are presented, as they never consciously experience these contents. Yet they demonstrate that they have considerable knowledge of these contents. Patients with neurotic-beliefs have knowledge that they just do not (cannot/ will not) believe. In addition, as for non-human animals, despite some claims to the contrary, it is more parsimonious to allow that they have first order knowledge simpliciter, without entailed belief and without knowing or believing that they know.

However, these cases raise two vital questions, which I will take up one at a time. First, why are we willing to attribute knowledge to these agents, but not beliefs? Are they meeting sufficient conditions for knowing, while they do not meet certain necessary conditions for believing? Velleman (personal communication 2007) suggests an answer regarding cases such as those detailed in this section:

> The subject's subjective probability for p is greater than his subjective probability for *not-p*, and this differential is reliably linked to the fact that p; but 1) subjective probability for p is not great enough to satisfy our intuitive threshold for all-out belief; and in some cases also 2) he misjudges the differential, claiming that he has no more credence in p than in *not-p* (a false second-order belief)...[Thus] we are willing to credit someone with knowledge on the basis of small differences in his cognitive states that *are* reliable indicators of the truth; but [these] are not sufficient [for the subject him/ herself] to qualify [for him/her] as beliefs.

While this answer does help to some extent, one is still left wondering why it is the case, that when one's subjective probability for p is greater than for *not-p* and this differential is reliably linked to the fact that p, our intuitive threshold for all-out belief is higher than that for knowledge. One possibility concerns the nature of belief, a cognitive attitude that aims constitutively at the truth (Velleman 2000, p.16), in contrast to the nature of knowledge, a factive attitude that could well be characterized as constitutively registering a truth rather than aiming at it. Understanding belief and knowledge in this way strongly suggests the possibility that some sort of registering of truth is an ontologically necessary precursor to aiming at the truth, as after all one must have some particular truth at which to aim.[38]

---

[38] However, there are two important things to note in this last sentence. First, consider that the phrase 'registering of truth' is not very specific. This is intended as indeed I am not claiming that in order to have a belief that p one needs to know p; I am making the far weaker claim that in order to have a belief that p, one must have knowledge of some q that is related in some non-trivial way to p. (See more on this below in the subsection 'The case for belief entailing knowledge.') Second, the phrase 'some sort of registering' is

The second important question raised by the analyses of these cases is: Why is it that the standard view in epistemology has been that knowledge entails belief, and that knowledge entails second-order knowing (both knowing that you know and knowing what you know)? It is because this dual entailment thesis, according to Jaakko Hintikka (1962), 'presuppose[s] a certain amount of rationality in the people whose attitudes are being discussed' (p.30). David Annis (1977) agrees that to hold that knowledge entails belief presumes rationality. However, Annis, unlike Hintikka, finds this view highly problematic: 'we cannot define knowledge by including rationality. Nor can we conditionalize the entailment thesis on the assumption of rationality' (p.223). To support his view he gives a counterexample in which rationality is not expected, and yet knowledge is still attributed: 'If we are told that the idiot savant does not believe, our reaction is not: If he does not believe, he must not really know; otherwise why would he not believe' (p.223). Rather, Annis points out, it is granted by many philosophers[39] that '...in such a case the person has knowledge' (p.223). Therefore, he concludes, if in cases such as this knowledge does not entail belief, knowledge need not entail belief. By adding many different cases to that of the savants, including those that arise in the real-world settings of cognitive psychology experiments and the clinical psychoanalytic situation,

---

meant to indicate that there are not only different levels of specificity of registration, but also different kinds of registerings. Do these match the different sorts of knowing?

Certainly against the view that knowledge is constitutively the registration of some truth p or some truth q related non-trivially to p, one might contend that while it is plausible for knowing-that, and maybe even probable for the discrimination and recognition types of knowledge, how could this account work for know-how and knowing-how-to, the dispositional and ability types of knowledge?

My reply must invoke truth registrations at the level of the brain—neuronal patterns involving motor and sensory cortical pathways interacting with 1) cerebellar input and feedback, and 2) brain areas associated with memory—along with more peripheral registrations at the level of spinal column, neuromuscular junction, and peripheral musculature. An example from baseball might help. What does it mean to have the know-how to hit a cut fastball? It means that one can reliably hit that type of pitch. Suppose B, after many failed attempts, finally does successfully hit a cut fastball. Consider this to constitute the first instance of truth registered; the truth in this case being the correct series of complicated perceptions and actions needed to accurately register and then respond to cut fastballs in order to hit them. Now, to the extent that B can repeat (perhaps tens of thousands of times) that particular complex entrainment of eyes, brain, hands, major muscle groups, in precisely the same truth registering-and-reacting pattern that has resulted in successfully hitting the cut fastball, to that extent B will eventually have the ability, i.e., the know-how, to hit that sort of pitch.

[39] Annis cites Ayer (1956, pp.32–35), Malcolm (1963, pp.226–228), and Unger (1967, pp.152–173) directly, and states there are others who hold this view.

the premise that there are instances of knowledge without entailed belief is broadened and strengthened. In addition, if this premise is strengthened, the conclusion, that knowledge can and does exist without belief, becomes all the more difficult to resist.

Unconscious knowledge/unconscious belief

Unconscious knowledge without unconscious belief

In the previous section, I presented several types of examples, all of which demonstrated first-order knowing without second-order knowing. In order to avoid later misunderstanding, and because it is a topic of general interest, let us at this point consider whether (and how) the phenomena of first- and second-order knowledge are related to those of first- and second-order consciousness.[40] Almost immediately it can be appreciated that although there is some area of overlap between first- and second-order knowledge and first- and second-order consciousness, there is no perfect one-to-one mapping. For example, when the winning-racehorse picker selects a winning horse, he is fully conscious of his choice: He is conscious of the specific horse he selects (first-order consciousness) and he can reflect both on the fact that he did make a choice and on his having chosen this particular horse (second-order consciousness). However, he has only first-order knowledge that the horse he picks is a winner. He does not know how he has made his choice; and especially early in his successful career, he does not know that he knows the winner. He has no second-order knowledge. This obtains for the chicken-sexer too. However, the situation is different for Jean (the French-Canadian 'student' of English history), the subjects in the subliminal and duck/rabbit experiments, the analytic patients drawing their dream elements, people with negative hallucinations, and savants. While these people also had first-order but no second-order knowledge, here even their first-order knowledge was unconscious.

Still, is it not the case that beliefs can be unconscious too? This leads to a very interesting set of arguments that developed among several philosophers

---

[40] These two types of consciousness have been known by various terms. For just a few examples: Ned Block (1991) refers to phenomenal and access consciousness, Gerald Edelman (1989) to primary and higher order consciousness, and David Rosenthal (1986) talks of HOTs or higher order thoughts to describe the consciousness of being conscious of something. Although I have lately favored 'primary consciousness' and 'reflective consciousness,' as this second term is quite descriptive, for the purpose of this chapter the terms first- and second-order consciousness work best as they avoid unnecessary confusion.

concerning Radford's (1966) claim that Jean, his fictional French-Canadian student of English history, unconsciously *knew*. Essentially Keith Lehrer (1970, 1974), Annis (1969), and Armstrong (1969–70, 1973) all argue that while Radford (1966) properly allows that Jean had unconscious knowledge, he illegitimately denies that he also had unconscious belief. Armstrong (1969–70, p.26) puts it thus: 'the case is a case of knowledge ...But...on the very same grounds that lead him to say it is a case of knowledge, he should say it is also a case of belief' (p.26). Lehrer (1970, p.137) further holds that Radford takes 'conscious conviction and a readiness to report as a condition of the application of the epistemic term [he] wish[es] to prove not to apply [i.e., belief] while rejecting these as conditions of the epistemic term [he] wish[es] to assume does apply [i.e., knowledge]' (p.137).

Radford (1970) addresses his critics: 'Having shown that Jean does not consciously believe that P, we are still, however, left with the possibility that he unwittingly, unconsciously believes this...But if our only reason for saying that Jean unwittingly believes that P were that he unwittingly knows that P, we should be assuming what is in question, *viz.*, that if someone knows that something is the case he therefore believes that something is the case' (p.105). Thus, unless it is accepted that knowledge necessarily entails belief, there is no reason to assume that Jean's unconscious knowledge entails his unconscious belief. Next, Radford (1970) gives a positive reason for denying that Jean has unconscious beliefs. He contrasts Jean's unconscious knowledge—immediately and simply obvious from his correct answers—with his putative unconscious belief, which as a 'theoretical construct' requires another level of inference (pp.106–107).

Note that if Radford's argument about Jean's having unconscious knowledge without unconscious belief holds, it will work for the other types of cases too. This is important because just as there are significant differences between knowledge and belief, there are also significant differences between unconscious knowledge and unconscious belief—the topic of the next subsection.

Differences between unconscious knowledge and unconscious belief

As is true regarding knowledge coming in many varieties (see the subsection on 'Various types of knowledge' above), there are several sorts of unconscious knowledge. On the simplest level, one can unconsciously discriminate between or among stimuli, as is true in the subliminal experiments. In addition, one can unconsciously know content, in the sense of being acquainted with it, as is demonstrated by the mere exposure effect and duck/rabbit experiments. Then there is unconsciousness with regard to know-how, both not being conscious of having know-how, and being unconscious with respect to how the know-how works. Savants, the chicken-sexer, and the winning-racehorse picker demonstrate both kinds of know-how unconsciousness; with consciousness of having the skill developing only with experience, while access to the nature of the skill[41] remains unconscious. Finally, one can be unconscious of knowing-that *p* in two different senses; unconscious about the knowing-that, and unconscious about the content, *p*.

Unconscious belief does not come in many types, only two. One can be unconscious of one's mental state of believing, perhaps mis-categorizing it as some other mental attitude. In addition, one can be unconscious about the contents of one's belief. Suppose that my mother is ill and I want very much for her to recover. At some point I might have a realistic belief that she is in fact dying. However, as this belief is one that is very painful, it might be the case that I repress this belief (i.e., its contents) and render it unconscious. Or, it might be that I am still conscious of the contents, but mis-type the mental attitude convincing myself that it is just a baseless fear that she is dying, a fear I can dismiss.

The priority of knowledge

The case for belief entailing knowledge

Much space in this chapter has been devoted to undermining the claim that knowledge entails belief (K → B). What if the entailment thesis went the other way such that belief entails knowledge (B → K)?[42] Peter Unger (1975/2002)

---

[41] That we categorize these feats as 'skills' presumes that there *is* a lawful manner in which the chicken-sexer, winning-racehorse picker, and savant each operate; just that in every case it is not known, maybe not even available to be known.

[42] According to Williamson (2000, pp.3, 41–48) even if knowledge does entail belief (and not vice versa), the conceptual independence of knowledge is not at stake. For example, even though every instance of being a dog entails having at least one dog-like quality, being a dog is conceptually prior to having at least one dog-like quality. (This example owes to Williamson, personal communication, 2006.)

Nonetheless, Williamson (2000) notes that the prevalent standard idea that knowledge is belief plus something else might in fact be due to the entailment thesis (K → B). In addition, he maintains that the conjunctive view of knowledge must be defeated in order to grant that knowledge is conceptually prior (p.48). He argues that this can be done rather simply. Just as red can not be analyzed as colored plus something else because the something else must include some specification of redness, knowledge cannot be analyzed as belief plus something else because the something else would have to include specifying knowledge in some way (Williamson 2000, pp.3,32).

makes such a claim, holding that for someone to have a reasonable belief one must have a reason for that belief, and this comes down to knowing something [43]—minimally a) some fact(s) and b) that the reason is connected to the belief (p.37). Oliver Johnson (1979) in a discussion of Unger's (1975/2002) book elaborates: 'If anyone gives, as his reason for believing X, some proposition "p", then for us to count p as a reason for him, and therefore to count the person reasonable in believing X for the reason p, he must *know* that p. Reasonable belief, it follows, entails knowledge' (p.379). Put another way, believing X (for any X) entails knowing that p (for some p related to X in the right way).

Zeno Vendler (1975) defends what at first glance seems to be a very specific, narrow, and limited case of belief entailing knowledge. Referring to the attitudes of a listener after a speaker has spoken, Vendler states, 'The knowledge of what one said does not imply belief, but the belief of what one said presupposes the knowledge of what one said' (pp.372–373). In other words, if Z says, 'I'm going to stop doing A right now,' in order for me to begin to asses whether or not to believe him as to whether or not he will stop doing A—i.e., to have a belief about this content—I have to know the content. While one might think that this pertains only to speech acts, upon reflection Vendler might have hit upon a general epistemological fact: In order to have any belief at all *about* some X, that X (or something non-trivially and predictably related to X) must be known, even if that knowledge is in the truth-registering sense of acquaintance or discrimination knowledge. Thereby belief entails knowledge, and not vice versa.

Samuel Guttenplan (1994) extends the idea of belief entailing knowledge to the idea that belief originated from knowledge. Like Williamson (2000) Guttenplan sees knowledge as a factive state that cannot be described as belief plus some other things. Instead, knowledge is central with belief 'as knowledge *minus* something' (p.297). He tells what he admits is a 'just so story' about some very early propositional attitude-using ancestors:

> [O]n seeing a spider, and also seeing A's extremely anxious-to-leave sort of behavior, it was natural to connect the two. What was said was that A feared the spider. And this kind of talk was itself built out of other kinds of relation between A and the spider: there was the 'seeing' relation...and of course there was the knowing relation. This latter was central to the functioning of the whole scheme: A had to be in that relation to the spider's presence for fearing...to so much as make sense. Now...this scheme had one great drawback: there were times when...a shadow on the wall provoked the

---

[43] Unger makes this point to support his argument that because reasonable belief entails knowledge, belief is no less susceptible than knowledge to skeptical arguments.

[spider] response…But of course this happened when in fact there was no spider… It was at this point that…someone suggested that a new attitude be invented, one which was exactly like knowledge in all but one respect: the requirement that things actually be as described…the new attitude was… 'quasi-knowledge'…[i.e., knowledge minus the spider's actual presence]…belief. (p.298)

The relationship of evidence to belief and knowledge

In the standard account, knowledge is belief plus something else. The view described in the 'just so story' above reverses this, holding that belief is knowledge minus something. Where does evidence fit in this equation both with respect to belief and knowledge? The standard analysis has it that belief plus evidence yields knowledge. But what if this were reversed too? Williamson (2000, pp.8–11, 184–186, 203–208) argues for this strongly, equating '…S's evidence with S's knowledge…$E = K$' (p.185). When it is the case that $E = K$, that one's evidence is equal to one's knowledge '…all one's knowledge serves as the foundation for all one's justified beliefs' (p.186). Filling this out: It is belief that gains grounds in its aim at the truth by adding evidence, and evidence is in the form of knowledge (p.208). Clearly, on this account (and related to Unger's claim described just above), a new equation: Belief plus Knowledge/Evidence yields Justified Belief, ($B + K/E = Justified\ B$), replaces the standard view equation: Belief plus Evidence yields Knowledge, ($B + E = K$).

The new equation fits the savant, chicken-sexer, and winning-horse picker cases quite naturally. The agents in these circumstances do not have beliefs about their capacities or about the outcome of a particular instance *until* they have established, through experience, that they know how to make these selections. On the basis of this K/E, namely, their experiential evidence that they have the know-how—they can form justified beliefs about their abilities and about the particulars of a specific chick or race.

The developmental priority of knowledge

Wimmer and Perner (1983) did a classic experiment that can be interpreted in a variety of ways, including one which suggests that children are demonstrably capable of knowing things before they can be shown to have beliefs. In the experiment, children were shown a puppet play in which a puppet boy named Maxi first puts some candies in a box and then goes out to play. While he is out playing the mother puppet moves the candies to the cupboard. Children are asked where Maxi will look for the candies on his return. Five-year-olds have no trouble indicating that Maxi will look for the candies in the box where he left them. However, three- and four-year-olds more often indicate that Maxi will look for the candies in the cupboard. These children, by virtue of their watching the play and seeing the puppet mother move the candies, *know* that the candies are in the cupboard, and this fact seems arresting. In the face of their own knowing, they seem unable to grasp that the other children could in fact not-know and thereby merely believe falsely.

This interpretation of this experiment may in itself not be convincing. However, let us add to it findings from non-human animals. Animals, functioning in ways that are adaptive, clearly possess knowledge, at least in the acquaintance, recognition, discrimination, and know-how senses, and probably in terms of knowing-that too. (For example, dogs know-that certain sounds are often associated with certain outcomes—cabinet door with dog biscuits, leash noises with going outside—and we can tell they know-that by their responsive behaviors.) However, could not one then assume that dogs (and other animals) also have beliefs? The answer is no. As Radford's argument made clear regarding inferring unconscious beliefs as well as unconscious knowledge in the case of Jean the French-Canadian student of English history, positing animal belief requires an additional level of inference over and above that which will suffice for animal knowledge.

Conclusions on the priority of knowledge

Each of the foregoing subsections takes up a different aspect of the priority of knowledge over belief. The subsection on belief entailing knowledge makes a case for knowledge being conceptually and ontologically fundamental. The subsection titled 'The relationship of evidence to belief and knowledge' presents the view that knowledge constitutes the evidence for belief, rather than the standard notion that in order to arrive at knowledge one needs belief plus evidence. Knowledge providing evidence for belief and not vice versa, amounts to a claim for knowing as the epistemologically prior state. Finally, the subsection on development considers that knowing is a state of mind available evolutionarily and developmentally earlier than believing.

Psychoanalysis and the priority of knowledge

This chapter has provided psychoanalytic data and theory in support of a radical view in epistemology and philosophy—that knowledge, rather than belief, is the fundamental epistemic mental state. Psychoanalytic data and theory have helped in two ways. First, to the question, 'but isn't it the case that knowledge entails belief?' psychoanalytic data provide answers favoring the independence of knowledge. Patients with negative hallucinations, for instance, clearly have unconscious contentful knowledge without any prior or concurrent beliefs about what they know. Further, neurotic patients (and most 'normal' people too) have neurotic-beliefs. These are actually phantasies, regarded as beliefs. Despite this, neurotic-beliefs, unlike beliefs-proper are not evidence sensitive. In fact neurotic-beliefs interfere with patients' use of knowledge as evidence. For example, some patients who are smart have neurotic-beliefs that they are dumb. Consequently, without outright denial of obvious evidential knowledge (such as intelligence quotient (IQ) tests and school performance) that confirm above average intellect, these patients isolate these facts. The knowledge of objectively measured intelligence, as is indicated by the IQ tests, etc., is intact, but inert; it is simply not believed. Thus, instead of having second-order true beliefs about knowing their intelligence, such patients continue with neurotic-beliefs about being dumb. The realm of their knowledge on this matter, and the realm of their beliefs are not just independent, but disconnected. Finally, the dream-drawing case illustrates another psychoanalytic situation in which contents are known in a first-order unconscious fashion without beliefs having played any role at all. In these ways psychoanalytic data help defeat the idea that knowledge entails belief (K → B).

Second, and perhaps more important, psychoanalytic theory has added something to the debate concerning first- and second-order knowledge—a debate compressed into the single question: 'If one knows mustn't one also know that (and what) one knows?'[44] Unconscious knowing, the existence of which is one of the most important assumptions of psychoanalysis, is also evinced in several of the cases demonstrating that one can indeed know without knowing one knows. It is *unconscious* knowledge that explains how Jean the French-Canadian knows but does not know he knows some English history. Unconscious knowledge also determines how the chicken-sexer can know males from females, and how the winning-racehorse picker can choose the winners, with neither practitioner having a clue how he knows, and at first, even that he knows. When we move beyond the constructed cases, unconscious knowledge figures just as importantly. The performances of savants, and the responses of subjects in mere exposure, subliminal, and duck/rabbit experiments, all illustrate agents knowing without knowing they know, all necessitating the posit of *unconscious* first-order knowledge. Finally, in examples involving actual psychoanalytic data too, cases such as negative hallucination and dream drawing, again first-order knowledge is shown to exist without second-order knowledge or second-order belief, with the first-order knowledge quite *unconscious.*

---

[44] There is also the related question, 'if one knows mustn't one also believe that (and what) one knows?'

In closing I shall remark that there is a significant way in which this chapter's contribution goes the other way too—by which I mean that the radical philosophical view that knowledge is the fundamental epistemological mental state points to a new understanding of the psychoanalytic endeavor itself. In order to illustrate this, let us return to Dr. N's negative hallucination. As he demonstrated with his manifest dream content, Dr. N had unconscious knowledge of my falling asleep. However, he had no conscious knowledge of my lapse. Even after I showed him the evidence of his dream he said, 'You did not fall asleep here last time! If you had, I'd be really furious.' However, I did, and so we have to assume that he was really furious, and that he rendered his fury unconscious too. What is the analytic task here? Certainly it is to make the unconscious conscious; to make content pertaining to my having fallen asleep and his feelings about it available to examine—this is vitally important. However, alone, this account is incomplete, and construes the analytic task too broadly and without the proper emphasis. More specifically, the analytic task goes deeper than generally facilitating a patient's possessing certain contents. In Dr. N's case it involves helping him know that he knew I fell asleep; helping him understand why, fearing his furious feelings, he had to try to un-know that knowledge. The compromising of one's knowledge and one's capacity to know, seen so clearly in negative hallucinations as a paradigmatic neurotic symptom, is arguably the most deleterious aspect of any neurosis, and it is present in every one. Keeping in mind the philosophical view of the primacy of knowledge can help analysts go beyond making the unconscious conscious toward making what *must be kept un-knowable* ultimately known.

References

Annis, D (1969). A note on Lehrer's proof that knowledge entails belief. *Analysis*, 29, 207–208.

Annis, D (1977). Knowledge, belief, and rationality. *The Journal of Philosophy*, 74, 217–225.

Armstrong, D (1969–70). Does knowledge entail belief? *Proceedings of the Aristotelian Society*, 7, 21–36.

Armstrong, D (1973). *Belief, Truth and Knowledge*. Cambridge, Cambridge University Press.

Ayer, A J (1956). *The Problem of Knowledge*. London, Penguin Books.

Block, N (1991). *Evidence against epiphenomenalism. Behavioral and Brain Studies*, 14, 670–672.

Brakel, LAW (1989). Negative hallucinations, other irretrievable experiences and two functions of consciousness. *The International Journal of Psychoanalysis*, 70, 461–479.

Brakel, LAW (1993). Shall drawing become part of free association? *Journal of the American Psychoanalytic Association*, 41, 359–394.

Brakel, LAW (2001). Phantasies, neurotic-beliefs, and beliefs-proper. *American Journal of Psychoanalysis,* **61**, 363–389.

Brakel, LAW (2009). *Philosophy, Psychoanalysis, and the A-Rational Mind.* Oxford, Oxford University Press.

Chambers, D and Reisberg, D (1985). Can mental images be ambiguous? *Journal of Experimental Psychology: Human Perception and Perfromance,* **11**, 317–328.

Chisholm, R (1957). *Perceiving.* Ithaca and London, Cornell University Press.

Danto, A (1968). *Analytical Philosophy of Knowledge.* Cambridge, Cambridge University Press.

Edelman, G (1989). *The Remembered Present: A Biological Theory of Consciousness.* New York, Basic Books.

Fisher, C (1957). Dreams and perceptions. *Journal of the American Psychoanalytic Association,* **2**, 389–445.

Freud, S (1900). *The Interpretation of Dreams.* Standard Edition, Vol. 4 & 5. Trans. and ed. J. Strachey. London, 1953, Hogarth Press.

Gettier, E (1963). Is justified true belief knowledge? *Analysis,* **23**, 121–123.

Goldman, A (1975). Innate knowledge. In Stephen Stich, ed. *Innate Ideas.* Chapter 6, 111–120. Berkeley, University of California Press.

Goldman, A (1976). Discrimination and perceptual knowledge. *The Journal of Philosophy,* **73**, 771–791.

Guttenplan, S (1994). Belief, knowledge, and the origins of content. *Dialectica,* **47**, 287–305.

Hartland-Swann, J (1958). *An Analysis of Knowing.* London, Unwin and Allen, New York, Macmillan.

Hintikka, J (1962). *Knowledge and Belief.* Ithaca, New York, Cornell University Press.

Johnson, O (1979). Ignorance and irrationality. *Philosophy Research Archives,* **5**, 368–417.

Jones, OR (1971). Knowing and guessing: by examples. *Analysis,* **32**,19–23.

Kim, J (1993). *Supervenience and Mind.* Cambridge, Cambridge University Press.

Kunst-Wilson, W and Zajonc, R (1980). Affective discrimination of stimuli that cannot be recognized. *Science,* **207**, 557–558.

Lehrer, K (1970). Believing that one knows. *Synthese,* **21**, 133–140.

Lehrer, K (1974). *Knowledge.* Oxford, Oxford University Press.

Lemmon, EJ (1967). If I know, do I know that I know? In Avrum Stroll, ed. *Epistemology: New Essays in the Theory of Knowledge.* New York, Harper and Row.

Lewis, D (1983). Mad pain and Martian pain. In David Lewis, ed. *Philosophical Papers, Volume 1,* 122–132. Oxford, Oxford University Press.

Lewis, D (1990). What experience teaches. In William Lycan, ed. *Mind and Cognition.* Oxford, Blackwell Press.

Macintosh, JJ (1979–80). Knowing and believing. *Proceedings of the Aristotelian Society,* **80**, 169–185.

Malcolm, N (1952). Knowledge and belief. *Mind,* **61**, 178–189.

Malcolm, N (1963). *Knowledge and Certainty.* Englewood Cliffs, NJ, Prentice Hall.

Mannison, DS (1976) 'Inexplicable knowledge' does not require belief. *The Philosophical Quarterly,* **26**, 139–148.

Margolis, J (1973). *Knowledge and Existence*. New York, Oxford University Press.

Pritchard, HA (1950). *Knowledge and Perception*. London, Oxford University Press.

Putnam, H (1975). *Mind, Language and Reality*. Cambridge, Cambridge Univeristy Press.

Radford, C (1966). Knowledge: By Examples. *Analysis*, **27**, 1–11.

Radford, C (1970). Does unwitting knowledge entail unconscious belief? *Analysis*, **30**, 103–107.

Reed, SK and Johnsen, JA (1975). Detection of parts in patterns and images. *Memory and Cognition*, **3**, 569–575.

Ring, M (1977). Knowledge: The cessation of belief. *American Philosophical Quarterly*, **14**, 51–59.

Rosenthal, D (1986). Two concepts of consciousness. *Philosophical Studies*, **40**, 329–359.

Ryle, G (1949). *The Concept of Mind*. Chicago, The University of Chicago Press.

Shevrin, H, Bond, J, Brakel, LAW, Hertel, R, and Williams, W (1996). *Conscious and Unconscious Processes*. New York, Guilford Press.

Shevrin, H, Snodgrass, M, Abelson, J, Kushwaha, R, and Brakel, LAW (in preparation). Unconscious facilitation and inhibition of phobic stimuli: N100 amplitude and latency moderate subliminal mere exposure effects.

Shope, R (1983). *The Analysis of Knowing*. Princeton, Princeton University Press.

Slap, J (1976). A note on the drawing of dream details. *Psychoanalytic Quarterly*, **59**, 455–456.

Stanley, J and Williamson, T (2001). Knowing how. *The Journal of Philosophy*, **98**, 411–444.

Stich, S (1978). Autonomous psychology and the belief-desire thesis. *The Monist*, **61**, 573–591.

Unger, P (1967). Experience and factual knowledge. *The Journal of Philosophy*, **64**, 152–173.

Unger, P (1975/2002). *Ignorance: A Case for Sceptism*. Oxford, Oxford University Press.

Velleman, JD (2000). *The Possibility of Practical Reason*. Oxford, Oxford University Press.

Vendler, Z (1975). On what we know. *Language, Mind and Knowledge. Minnesota Studies in the Philosophy of Science*, **7**, 370–390.

Williamson, T (2000). *Knowledge and Its Limits*. Oxford, Oxford University Press.

Wimmer, H and Penner, J (1983). Beliefs about beliefs: representations and constraining functions of wrong belief in young children's understanding of deception. *Cognition*, **13**, 103–128.

Wittgenstein, L (1953). *Philosophical Investigations*. New York, Macmillan.

Woozley, AD (1953). Knowing and not knowing. *Proceedings of the Aristotelian Society*, **53**, 151–172.

Part III

Vagueness and a–rationality

Epistemology, metaphysics, philosophy of mind

Chapter 3

The limits of rationality: Vagueness, a case study

Introduction

What is vagueness: Examples

Vagueness is a topic that has been of interest to philosophers since ancient times. Perhaps the simplest way to understand vagueness is by first presenting two of the most common examples of concepts that are considered paradigmatically vague: 1) baldness and 2) heaps, which both involve the 'sorites paradox,' which will also be demonstrated just below. Thus, if a totally bald man with no hair at all gains one hair, is he still bald or not bald? What about two hairs? Bald of course, because what difference does one hair make, or two? But what about iterating this many times, single hair by single hair until the man has a full head of hair? At what point did he go from bald to not bald? Which hair made the difference? The sorites paradox of the heap is similar. This time let us start with a heap of sand. Take one grain away—do you still have a heap or is this a non-heap? Of course it is still a heap. But what about after two grains are removed, and three, and n, $n + 1$, $n + 2$? Which number of grains n, $n + 1$, $n + 200$, etc., marks the difference between heap and non-heap? The sorites paradox of baldness and heaps demonstrates that the concepts of baldness and heaps are vague concepts—in each it cannot be precisely specified as to what is and what is not in its extension. (In psychology terms: The categories of baldness and heaps are not precise because one cannot precisely determine what is and what is not a member of these categories.)

Rationality yields paradox

The paradoxical nature of vagueness is not fully captured by the fact of vague extensions (memberships) or of vague concepts/categories. Concepts without sharp boundaries and categories with borderline members are not in themselves paradoxical. Rather, a paradox (over and above the sorites paradox) arises over puzzling outcomes that occur when reasoning of a highly rational sort is used in trying to understand vague concepts. Thus it is sound and rational to reason that if a single grain of sand is removed from a heap, it will still be a heap; a grain of sand is so small. Further, it is rational to conclude that if two grains are removed it will still be a heap. After all, one grain of sand is very similar to two grains of sand. Likewise, what remains following the loss of two grains is highly similar to what remains after the loss of one grain. If removing one grain leaves the heap intact as a heap, so will removing two. It is also entirely rational to generalize: if a heap continues as a heap after the removal of n grains, it will do so after the removal of $n + 1$ grains, and that if this is true for one iteration, it must be true for any number $(n, n + 1, n + 2, …)$ of iterations. And yet, after some finite number of grains is removed, some $n + 1$ grains, it is rational to accept that no heap remains even when it had been rational to conclude that there was still a heap after the removal of n grains. So, finally, it is rational to conclude, that despite sound reasoning throughout, with no step a misstep, something has gone wrong; and this is the paradox!

A-rationality emerges

What has gone wrong with the rational reasoning in the above examples? Can it be that one grain is not similar to two; or that n grains are not similar to $n + 1$? Or maybe the sand pile minus n grains is not similar to that which remains when $n + 1$ grains are removed? No, not at all likely. Perhaps other aspects of the process of generalization are to be faulted, such that what is true for grain number one and grain number two will not work for grains n and $n + 1$? Again, no. Could it possibly be that there is something wrong with *modus ponens*—if p then q, where if p is true q will be true too? No. Or, less implausibly, maybe the situation has been improperly set up. Let us check: Let p be 'H minus n grains is a heap.' Let q be 'H minus $n + 1$ grains is a heap.' No, there seems to be nothing wrong with the set-up here: if p is true, it is the case that 'H minus n grains is a heap'; then q will be true too as indeed it will be the case that 'H minus $n + 1$ grains is a heap' also. In short, there is no problem at all with any of this very rational reasoning—but it leads to paradox.

Moreover, as I maintain in this chapter, this paradox[1] itself leads to a further paradox—namely, in the very attempts to fully rationalize vague concepts and their attendant paradoxes, it is *a-rationality* that clearly (and surprisingly) emerges. Now, before this thesis can be demonstrated, or even fully elaborated, there are many tasks ahead. I will first need to set out the basics of a-rationality, and in particular the characteristics and operating principles that differentiate it from both irrationality and rationality. Then, various philosophical views of vagueness will be addressed, with an emphasis on how several of the treatments

---

[1] The paradox again being that despite many steps, all with flawless reasoning, wrong outcomes result.

eventuate in *a-rational* outcomes. This takes us through the next two sections on 'A-rationality: General considerations' and 'Vagueness: General considerations,' respectively. Then the following two sections, investigating vagueness from another angle, are devoted to the metaphysical aspects of both a-rationality and vagueness. They are titled 'A-rational objects' and 'Ontic vagueness.' I close the chapter with the final section, 'Conclusions.'

A-rationality: General considerations

A brief look at rationality and then irrationality—two modes of thinking from which a-rationality differs substantially—will prove helpful in appreciating the unique nature of a-rationality.

Rational thinking

Human beings, it is widely held, have the capacity for rational thinking. Although we seldom function as perfectly rational agents, our ordinary behavior is considered largely rational, in an everyday way. For example, we do often have at least some knowledge of what we want—ranging from the very concrete satisfaction of our needs/desires to the very abstract notion of how we would like to conceive of ourselves—and some beliefs about what would be required to get what we want. We consider our options along many dimensions; e.g., the feasibility of this versus that plan; the consequences of each individually and comparatively, both for ourselves and for others; and short-term payoffs and costs as opposed to long terms benefits, etc.

In order for an agent to count as rational and for an act to be rational, several constraints must be in place.

1. Rational agents cannot hold any belief as a belief when they are simultaneously aware of some compelling evidence against the belief; and such agents must be able to evaluate evidence for or against beliefs independently of wishes and desires. When evidence shows that a belief cannot be true, although its content can still be present in a phantasy or daydream and it can likewise remain part of what is wished for or desired, a rational agent can no longer *believe* that content. Psychoanalysts term the evaluation of beliefs with respect to available evidence 'reality testing,' a set of skills developing as we mature. Even in adults reality testing is a capacity often interfered with, and for many reasons.

2. Rational agents, to the extent they are truly acting rationally, also strive to remain largely consistent, avoiding conflicts between beliefs and even sometimes between desires. Thus, if I believe it is hot and raining in Ann Arbor now, I cannot also believe that it is cold and snowing in Ann Arbor now. If I want the tuna rare, I cannot also want it well done. Less strictly, but still worth mentioning, there are incompatible desires that the rational thinker must recognize as problematic and work toward resolving. If I desire to go to Australia this summer and at the same time

want to stay home, I have got some thinking to do. Perhaps more interestingly, the rational agent tries to be consistent and avoid conflicts with regard to his/her self-concept. Thus if my colleague has a picture of himself as stingy, he will have to square that view with his frequent generous offers of time and sizeable donations to his preferred political candidate.

3. Related to both above, rational agents to the extent they are rational do not tolerate contradictions. If I am rational and assert that it is the case that that tie is red, I cannot also assert that it is not the case that the tie is red. If I say that it is true that I am hungry, angry, sleepy, I cannot then also claim that I am not hungry, angry, sleepy.

4. Rational agents can use indexicals regarding person, time, and place 'properly'—in other words, agents operating rationally can readily distinguish self from others, here from any number of theres, and now (present) from various thens (both past and future).

These four constraints of everyday rationality are in accord with what we might regard as basic principles of everyday logic, which include the ascription of 'true' or 'false' to various propositions; the law of non-contradiction; the law of the excluded middle; and grounding oneself and one's statements in time, place, and person.

Irrationality

Irrationality is not simply thinking without the constraints enumerated above; it is any of 1) rational thinking gone astray, *violating* the everyday principles of logic, 2) rational thinking put to irrational, deleterious ends, 3) a-rational thinking put to irrational ends, or 4) some combination. As I show in the next subsection, a-rationality is a form of thinking that operates *outside* (rather than in violation) of rationality and its principles. Hence this distinction is important.

For a demonstration of irrationality, let us take a patient who comes into psychoanalytic treatment with two primary symptoms—premature ejaculations and a fear of elevators. Early in his analysis he adds that he also feels nervous about cans with open jagged edges, has worries about falling into manholes, and is anxious about animal traps in the woods near his suburban neighborhood. Although any of these *might* cause an injury, he knows it is irrational to live in fear of any of these. Moreover he *knows* rationally that even elevators are quite safe. Certainly his evidential experience suggests the same; and thus his fear of elevators puts him at odds with major aspects of his self-concept. Nonetheless, he acts as though he had the belief that elevators are dangerous. This belief, defying as it does reality testing, is not just false; it is faulty and irrational; it is a 'neurotic-belief.'[2]

---

[2] 'Neurotic-belief' is a term I have used for such faulty beliefs. I have suggested that neurotic-beliefs operate not as beliefs–proper, but instead as phantasies—phantasies that are treated

Looking at this patient's other symptom, premature ejaculation, a similar situation obtains. He *knows* that vaginas are not dangerous; and yet despite evidence to the contrary and despite the bad effect the symptomatic solution of premature ejaculation has had on his self-concept (and his sexual life), the analyst can infer that the patient unconsciously holds a neurotic-belief to the effect that vaginas are indeed frightening places. Why is this inference justified? Because, rational assessment notwithstanding, the patient *acts* in accord with an irrational and unconscious neurotic-belief having 'dangerous vagina' as part of its content.[3]

There is another part to this story. Using his capacity for rational thinking, but toward the symptom's irrational ends, this patient finds evidence for his fears. He uses the Google search engine and comes up with several cases of people hurt in elevator accidents, particularly in elevators having overactive doors. He rationally 'rationalizes' his premature ejaculation symptom too; he is often in a hurry during the sex act; his partner has made aggressive comments toward him; and she does have some character traits that could be perceived as emasculating.

Thus with this patient we can see 1) his rational view of elevators, women, and himself—consistent, evidence based, reality tested; 2) his irrational neurotic-beliefs, in which the principles of everyday logic are abrogated; and 3) aspects of rational thinking appropriated by the irrational symptoms as he attempts to 'rationalize' his irrational symptoms. In addition, as we see in the next subsection, that is not all. His thinking and his symptoms also demonstrate a-rational mentation.

A-rationality

Unlike irrationality, a-rationality is not rationality gone awry. Rather, a-rationality might be characterized as 'the not-yet rational'—this, both in the sense that a-rationality is a form of mentation routinely employed by very young humans, and arguably it is a mode of mentation utilized by a great variety of non-human animals. (See Brakel and Shevrin 2003.) A-rationality has

---

as beliefs-proper, taking on some of the functional roles of beliefs-proper. This is all to the detriment of their holders. (Neurotic-beliefs are discussed briefly in Chapter 2, but for a much fuller account see Brakel, 2001, 2009, particularly Chapter 7.)

[3] At some point in the analysis as it progresses, the analyst will be able to suggest that such an unconscious phantasy is quite central in the patient's symptomatic behavior. In addition, after learning more details, the analyst will be able to make a further and more precise inference about the nature of the 'dangerous' vaginas feared by the patient and relate this to his other symptom(s). This connection is presented to the reader in the next subsection of this chapter.

been most extensively characterized by Freud. As early as 1900 he elaborated two very different types of mentation. One type, that consisting of the ordinary everyday logic of our (mostly) rational thoughts, he termed 'secondary process' mentation. The other type, 'primary process' mentation, he found to predate and then co-exist with the secondary processes, operating not only routinely in young children, but also in the dreams, daydreams, and psychological symptoms of adults (and children), sometimes quite unconsciously.

The primary processes (of mentation), as posited by Freud (1900), have both negative and positive characteristics. On the negative side, the primary processes *lack* (rather than violate) the principles of everyday logic that are hallmarks of typical (mostly) rational ordinary human thought. So, primary process mentation takes place with no conception of past or future; there is only a tenseless, unexamined present. Further, in primary process thinking there is no reality testing; no attempt to regulate representations for considerations of truth. Further, as Anna Freud (1936, p.7) added, in primary process thought, '...opposites are not mutually exclusive and may even coincide.' Taken together, it is not surprising that in primary process thought standard logic is not operative. Notably the law of the excluded middle is not in place and, contradictions, which are not even understood as such, are 'tolerated.' For example, if there are not yet any notions of truth or falsity, and if opposites are not mutually exclusive, it is clear that the primary process-thinker is not in any position to evaluate propositions with respect to each of them being either true or false. Following from this, contradictions (all of which are unrecognized) abound, unregulated. As I have explained elsewhere (Brakel 2002, p.2, n.2):

> ...before attempts to regulate representations for considerations of truth, any proposition that is considered merely 'is.' While an external view would regard this as a default consideration-as-true, from the internal viewpoint there is no attempt or even capacity to get the truth conditions right. That being the case, take some X that 'is' (i.e., is considered-true); but if a contradiction of this X is also regarded in just the same manner, this ~X, prior to considerations of truth and falsity, 'is' (i.e., is considered-as-true) no less.

A similar point can be made with respect to tenselessness: 'If every moment is an unexamined timeless present, a "now" with no history and no future, X held at moment t will not be negated by ~X being held at $t + 1$.'[4]

On the positive side, primary process mentation is characterized by two central principles—displacement and condensation (Freud, 1900)—both

---

[4] I owe this last point to Jennifer Church (personal communication) and have used it in a prior article: Brakel 2002, p.2, n2.

operating on the basis of *associative connections*. In condensation, multiple contents (ideas, images, thoughts, words, etc.) become associatively linked and are then represented by a single content or even a part of one. Elements that are *similar* in any one of a whole variety of ways tend to become associatively linked. For example, if two items are contiguous in time or space, they can be represented together. In addition, elements become associated—leading to a single condensed representation—if they share a feature, even a quite inessential one, and/or if they resemble each other in peripheral, global, significant, or insignificant ways, along any dimension including both physical resemblance, and functional equivalence. Note that these resemblances can be quite subjective and idiosyncratic.

Displacements are condensations in reverse. In displacements one element associated with another represents it and is a substitute for it. Examples of displacements are parts standing for wholes, and tokens standing for types. As with condensations, the associative grounds for displacements are rather fluid: one content can be displaced onto another if they are contiguous in time or space; and/or if the two are *similar* in any of the great many ways elaborated above for condensations. Primary process mentation, in addition to having condensation and displacement as organizing principles, also is marked by a 'ready tendency' for the associative connections producing both condensation and displacement (Brenner 1955/1974, p.51).[5]

The role of similarity in a-rationality

Similarity is an essential (perhaps the essential) relation in a-rationality. To illustrate let us return to the patient with premature ejaculations, an elevator phobia, and the ancillary symptoms: anxiety about cans with jagged openings, fears of falling into manholes, and nervousness regarding animal traps near his home. Remember that the patient came to treatment understanding that despite his attempts at rationalizations, all of these symptoms were largely irrational. Thus, when in the course of the treatment, the analyst is able to make the interpretation that the patient has been long holding onto an unconscious phantasy that vaginas are dangerous places, the patient can readily appreciate how maintaining this phantasy could very well play an important causal role in his premature ejaculation symptom. But what can this central interpretation tell us (and the patient) about the elevator phobia and all the secondary fears? In addition, is there any way that the patient's fear of vaginas be specified more precisely?

---

[5] Examples of displacements and condensations follow in the next several subsections.

By understanding the role of similarity in a-rational mentation the ancillary symptoms can be shown to make sense, and a much more detailed and specific grasp of the vagina fear can be provided. Elevators, jagged can openings, manholes, and animal traps are all *similar* in that they are apertures with features potentially dangerous to a limb or member of a person's body. Vaginas do not usually belong in this category. However, if one has the unconscious phantasy/neurotic-belief that a vagina has teeth (vagina dentate), it fits very well. A vagina with teeth might harm a man's penis as he penetrates, just as an elevator door might close on a person's leg, or a jagged can opening could hurt someone's finger. With a manhole, someone could fall down and be hurt, and an animal trap, perhaps most resembling the feared phantasied vagina dentate, could tear and bloody a foot or ankle. Note that while all of these fears are irrational, they are also all *a-rationally* similar, belonging to the primary process category 'openings that are dangerous to a man and have features that could trap and hurt various of his members.' Relatedly, while the symptoms themselves are incontestably irrational, much of the thinking involved in their construction is neither rational nor irrational—but a-rational—with the a-rationally based categorizations appropriated to the irrational ends of the symptom.

A-rational/primary process types of categorizations can be in the service of goals that are not irrational in the least, for instance, in original solutions to problems and in various creative endeavors. In fact, I suggest later in the chapter that some philosophers grappling with the problem of ontic vagueness have come up with solutions that are predicated on a-rational principles. First though, in the following, I provide some brief examples of a-rationality, demonstrating its prominent presence in a wide range of mental events, some far afield from neurotic symptoms.

Examples

A-rationality in dreams   Dreams show a number of primary process a-rational features. Recently (August 2008) I had the following dream: 'Barack Obama is a woman, *and* he is just as he is, a man. Also he/she is my friend.' In the dream there is no negation. It cannot be the case that Obama is both now a woman and just as he is, and yet the dream has it that he is both man and woman with no need to negate either state or statement. There is no law of excluded middle. In the dream that Obama is a man does not imply that he is not a woman; nor does Obama's being a woman imply that Obama is not a man. My initial association to the 'man and woman' part of the dream immediately lead to thoughts of Hillary Clinton, the other Democrat making a strong showing in the 2008 race for the presidency. Combining both of them suggests that the primary process mechanism of condensation was also operative in this dream.

In another dream, I dreamt that 'Ernie, the character from Sesame Street, is alive and well.' In this dream, Ernie, the muppet, is a displacement from my late Uncle Ernie, whom I miss and who I wish were alive and well. This dream also demonstrates an unexamined present, a feature of many dreams, where the past is relived as if ongoing. Person and place indexicals are also often rearranged in dreams; one location can be misrepresented by another associated with it, and, more strikingly, the dreamer's own agency can be experienced through another dream figure.[6]

A-rationality in children's everyday thoughts A toddler looks out the window, and although it is clearly raining, he says, 'The sun, see (pointing). Go park!' The child is not crazy; rather he was told that if the sun came out later, he could be taken to the park. Here, in the interest of a wish to go to the park, he confuses the past (when there was sun) and future (when there probably will be sun) with the sun-less present. He makes the present more to his liking. This is possible because at this stage the child does not regulate his cognitive attitudes in terms of truth considerations. He might say that it is true that it is raining *and* that the sun is out. He might say that he cannot say whether or not it is true that it is raining, etc.

Children also frequently generalize on the basis of inessential parts, as for instance, when they consider all four-legged animals 'doggies' because dogs are the animals most familiar to them. Similarity assessment on the basis of inessential parts is one the most important types of a-rationally mediated categorizations, the topic addressed next.

A-rational categorizations There are many types of a-rationally based primary process categories. These include categories formed associatively on the basis of superficial similarity, and those based on the similarity of inessential parts. Poets (and others) can use such a-rational categories for similes and metaphors. For example, Shakespeare can ask, 'shall I compare thee to a summer's day?' Similarly Robert Burns can proclaim, 'My love is like a red red rose.'[7] Further, birds (and other animals) can use a-rationally based categories for successful foraging. They tend to return to areas sharing some common

---

[6] For more on a-rationality, particularly with respect to agency in dreams, see the section '"Me" in dreams' in Chapter 4 of this volume.

[7] For an example of an a-rational category producing a metaphor, consider the following lines from Fernando Pessoa's sonnet, 'Ah! A sonnet': 'My heart is just a crazy admiral who's abandoned his career at sea.' (translated by Arthur Brakel).

small visual features associated with the best places to feed. Hummingbirds, for instance, choose fluted shapes of an orange-red shade. A-rational categories predicated on associative similarities also include family resemblance classifications of all sorts; categories formed owing to common functional roles of their members; and categories arrived at because of a mood or feeling state of being aroused. An instance of this last type can be seen in my friend Z. He experiences a very distinct and unique feeling of nostalgia whenever he views any Expressionist painting, smells a particular aroma (wood burning), or comes across a stray cat. Based upon the unique feeling any one (or some combination) of these seemingly disparate items occasions, they form for Z an a-rationally based primary process category.

A-rationality in classical conditioning   A classically conditioned animal salivates at the ringing of a bell because in the past that bell tone has preceded the appearance of food. Whenever this sort of classical conditioning is successfully established, the animal is operating under mentation best described as a-rational. The salivating is initially the unconditioned response. Later it becomes also the conditioned response, as it occurs whenever the conditioned stimulus, the bell tone, sounds. Certainly such a response is not rational or irrational; it is a-rational, as it has been conditioned owing to the bell tone's *contiguity in time* with the unconditioned stimulus—the food. Now suppose that the experimenter wants the conditioned stimulus to generalize. The stimuli for which this will work will be those that are *similar* to the bell in various *a-rational primary process ways*. Some such stimuli will be similar to the bell in time—i.e., just before the bell; others will be similar in place—perhaps a light will go on at the same time as the bell. If the animal has seen the bell apparatus, perhaps an apparatus that looks like it, even if it makes no sound will be similar enough to produce the conditioned response. Conversely, an apparatus that looks quite different but produces the same or a similar sound could also produce the conditioned response and function as a generalized conditioned stimulus.[8]

A-rationality in psychotic symptoms   As is true for neurotic symptoms, psychotic symptoms too demonstrate much a-rational/primary process mentation. A patient with chronic schizophrenia, Mrs. M, had an acute relapse of her psychosis after having been diagnosed with an advanced and painful gynecological malignancy. Before we could achieve an adequate dosage of antipsychotic medication, the patient was behaving in the following way: She was pushing a bottle of 'Head and Shoulders' brand shampoo into and away from

---

[8] For additional material on a-rationality and conditioning see the penultimate section in Chapter 5 of this volume.

her pelvic area and screaming 'delivery of the head and shoulders is killing me.' Mrs. M was hallucinating and the content pertained to events some decades past when she was delivering her children. Many aspects of a-rationality are demonstrated with this example. The patient was living in an unexamined (wishful) present of many years earlier such that her current tumor pain could be associated, condensed, and ultimately conflated with the pain of the long-ago childbirths. The heads and shoulders of her children were displaced upon the shampoo bottle, which not only had a head and shoulder shape, but also was actually called 'Head and Shoulders.' This displacement entailed a-rational categorizing: the shampoo, a-rationally categorized, was not classified as it would have been rationally along with other soaps or body care products. Instead, particularly given the product's name and the shape of the bottle, it was associated with specific body parts of her not-yet born children, and categorized just as would be actual body parts.

Summary of the defining features of a-rationality

Before moving on to describe vagueness, this is a good time to review the hallmarks of a-rationality as have been described.

In terms of positive characteristics, a-rational (or primary process) mentation is marked by mental attitudes and contents formed by (or at very least strongly influenced by) the operation of two mental processes, displacement and condensation. The displacements and condensations function on the basis of associative links predicated on various sorts of similarity relations, specifically those that are not rationally based. These include contiguity in space and time; similarity of functional parts; and similarity among superficial, small, or inessential features.

On the negative side, a-rational mentation does not function under the laws of common sense logic. Different from violating these laws (as is the case for irrationality), in a-rational mentation the law of the excluded middle is not in operation, and negations and contradictions are not recognized and in this sense 'tolerated.' A-rational mentation is mentation that is 'not-yet rational,' hence considerations of truth or falsity do not apply. In addition, time is experienced as an unexamined present, there is no consistent univocal agency, and place is subject to here/there ambiguities.

***

If this chapter is to be successful, I will have to make the case that aspects of vagueness (and/or attempts at solutions to vagueness problems) actually belong in the previous subsection, in which examples of a-rationality are described. In order to do this, I will first have to give at least a rough account of several views of vagueness, each attempting to grapple with its paradoxes.

Next, I will need to demonstrate what in each of these attempts leads to outcomes that look surprisingly a-rational. Hence let us proceed to the section on 'Vagueness: General considerations.'

Vagueness: General considerations

The role of similarity in vagueness

Although the similarity relation plays a different role in vagueness than it does in a-rationality, in both phenomena relations of similarity are central. First of all, 'similarity' itself is vague and is easily caught up in a sorites paradox of its own. Is this coffee cup, A, similar to this other one, B? Well, they are the same color, shape, weight, texture, and have the same logo; so yes, they are similar. But what if we were to take one molecule from A and give it to B? Are they still similar? Sure, what difference will one or two molecules make? However, let us keep doing that with one molecule at a time, iterated many, many times. Are cups A and B still similar after the transfer of 40,000 molecules? Or are A and B now different? What about when all the molecules of A have been transferred to B? Now they do not seem similar at all, with A having no mass (and no existence) and B having twice that of the original cup. But what was the dividing line between similar and different; at which molecule transfer did A stop being similar to B and begin to be not-similar, i.e., different? The similarity relation is without a doubt indeterminate and vague.

Additionally, similarity figures essentially in any sorites paradox and therefore in the phenomenon of vagueness generally. Let us return to the familiar case of baldness. If a man with a full head of hair loses one hair is he bald or not bald? What about two hairs? Not bald, of course. However, now repeat this many times single hair by single hair until the man has no hair at all. At what point did he go from not-bald to becoming bald? Which hair made the difference? Really, this sort of paradox is predicated on the strength of two interlocking *similarity* relations: that between n hairs and $n + 1$ hairs and that between the head of hair minus n hairs and minus $n + 1$ hairs. However, note that the similarities here are both vague (as above) and non-transitive. (While n may be very similar, almost identical, and certainly indiscriminable from $n + 1$, which is almost identical and indiscriminable from $n + 2$, etc., and so forth, n is quite different from $n + 1,000,000$).[9] Of course the same two similarity relations hold in every other sorites paradox case. Given a heap of sand, take grains away one at a time. Which number of grains, n, $n + 1$, $n + 200$, etc., marks the difference

---

[9] See Dummett (1975/1997, p.111) for more on non-transitivity and 'not discriminably different.'

between heap and non-heap? If $n + 200$ is suggested, the extreme similarity both of the sand pile minus $n + 200$ to the sand pile minus $n + 199$ grains, and that of $n + 200$ to $n + 199$ casts doubt on this solution. Hence the paradox, and hence the pivotal role of similarity.

Views on vagueness

Epistemic view

The epistemic view of vagueness, perhaps best explicated by Timothy Williamson (1994) and Roy Sorensen (2001), holds that vagueness derives from the combination of our representational systems, our competence therewith, and our ignorance. Most readily illustrated by those cases involving unclear boundaries (as with the baldness, heap, and similarity examples above), the epistemic view insists that there *are* sharp boundaries among bald, not bald, and hairy; among similar, not similar, and different; and between some collection being a heap or not. Further and consequently, those philosophers holding the epistemic view assert that there *is* a single grain added that makes a collection a heap and a single hair removed making a man bald. It is just the case that we can never know which hair or grain it is ($n - 1$, or n, or $n + 1$, or $n + 1000$) that will constitute the boundary. Note that on this view of vagueness our not knowing will not be due to incompetence with any of the concepts involved (heaps, collection, boundaries, similarity, difference, baldness, etc.). Moreover there is no additional information that would help; we will not know because we cannot know—the precise boundary is unknowable.[10]

A-rational analog   So what is a-rational in this solution? On the face of it, nothing. However, there is a deep analogy. A-rational/primary process thinkers cannot distinguish between concepts that rational thinkers distinguish readily. For example, take frogs. Presumably, when exposed to small black objects of a certain size, they have a reflex capture and swallow reaction. They do this whether these black objects are metal BB pellets or bugs, no matter how

---

[10] For Williamson (1994, pp.237–244), our ignorance regarding vagueness is a species of inexact knowledge—inexact knowledge that cannot be made more exact. Suppose we were to claim that it is removing the—99th hair that constitutes the border between not bald and bald. We would no more have the right to claim that we *knew* this than we would if we contended that we knew (by observation) that there were 100,704 people in the Michigan Stadium on a particular football Saturday. Even if we were correct about the number of people in the stadium, Williamson maintains that since we cannot distinguish by observation 101,704 from 101,703, we cannot claim to know. (Could Wiilliamson's view accommodate an observational savant who could accurately and reliably distinguish 101,704 from 101,703? I owe this question to Arthur Brakel.)

much exposure and training frogs have both with the BBs and with bugs. Frogs, seemingly, have a concept roughly described as 'black object' that *cannot* be better differentiated. (See Millikan 1993, p.75.) On the epistemic view of vagueness, we rational/secondary process thinkers are like the a-rational thinking frogs insofar as we cannot make precise distinctions regarding concepts that are vague for us—such as bald/not bald/ hairy; heap versus not a heap; tall/not tall/short; similar/not similar/different, etc.

Many-valued logic, degrees of truth, and supervaluation views

Vagueness introduces problems for standard logic. Contradictions abound when two-valued logic and bivalence (i.e., law of excluded middle)—something is true or else it is false—are applied to vague predicates, properties, or objects. Willard V.O. Quine (1981) states the problem thus: '...if the loss of a hair makes no man bald, then neither does the loss of any number of them. Bivalence seals the paradox, requiring as it does at each stage that the statement that...the man is bald, be univocally true or false' (p.91). As a possible solution Quine notes that stipulating boundaries could work to obviate vague problems arising from cases like baldness and heaps; but as he readily acknowledges, this move has deeper problems than mere inelegant arbitrariness.[11] Citing Peter Unger's (1979b) work (discussed later in this chapter), in which a table is dismantled molecule by molecule, Quine asks, '...when is a table not a table? No stipulations will avail us here, however arbitrary' (1981, p.92).

Attempts to deal with the problem of bivalence in the face of vagueness have lead to various introductions of a third category in addition to something being either true or false. This takes a few different forms: 'neither true nor false'; 'true to such-and-such degree' (Williamson, 1994, p.96); and 'supervaluations,' in which each and every sharpening of a vague predicate is evaluated such that '...a sentence is true iff [if and only if] it is true on all precisifications, false if false on all precisifications, and neither true nor false otherwise' (Keefe and Smith 1997, p.23). These supervaluations are then definitely true, definitely false, or indefinite, respectively. Each of these postulates of a third category has a number of proponents motivated by differing concerns.[12]

---

[11] As an extreme measure, arbitrary stipulations might even be applied for setting a boundary between childhood and adulthood, and declaring at what stage in embryologic development mammalian life begins, etc. However, I share Quine's qualms and, with him, conclude that this is hardly a satisfying solution.

[12] Michael Tye (1994/1997) developed a three-valued logic; Kenton Machina (1976/1997) and Dorothy Edgington (1992/1997) are degree theorists; and Henryk Mehlberg (1958/1997) and Kit Fine (1975/1997) are supervaluationists.

However, all of these three-category solutions suffer from another feature of vagueness—namely that vagueness versus preciseness is itself vague, which leads to second-order (and higher order) vagueness. (See Sorensen 1985, pp.134–137.) Here is how this plays out. Just as it is hard to draw a distinct line between bald and not bald and between not bald and hairy, it is difficult to decide the sharp boundaries among 1) bald and borderline bald, 2) borderline bald and borderline not bald, 3) borderline not bald and not bald, 4) not bald and borderline hairy, and 5) between borderline hairy and hairy. Hence, just as ascriptions of true or false will have borderline cases, so will the evaluation of 'neither true nor false.' Borderline cases will result. Similarly, degrees of truth will be infected with the same sort of problem. Just as there are borderline cases of complete truth there will be borderline cases of particular degrees of truth. Finally, for supervaluations, since what counts as an 'admissible precisification' is vague, and 'all precisifications' must be evaluated, there will be cases of indefinitely true, indefinitely false, and even indefinitely indefinite statements. (Sorensen, 2001, p.55).

A-rational analog   Attempts to deal with the contradictions that arise regarding vague concepts introduce solutions that look very much like a-rational/primary process thinking. For example, the many-valued logics in allowing that something can be neither true nor false operate outside the law of the excluded middle. To this extent many-valued logics operate in the same way that a-rational thinking does. Interestingly, Graham Priest (1985–86, p.101) in attempting to solve the problem of contradictions and multi-valued logics takes yet a further step in the primary process/a-rational direction, as he seems to welcome contradictions. He says:

> Given two states of affairs, then there are, in general, four possibilities. The first may hold but not the second, the converse may obtain, both may hold, or neither may hold. Thus, for a given assertion, A, we might expect these four possibilities for the two states of affairs: *A is true* and *A is false.* The received theory assumes that only two of the four possibilities may arise. [Namely that the first may hold but not the second, or the converse.] Slightly more liberal views allow that a third may occur, that A is neither true nor false. If nothing else symmetry suggests that the fourth should be countenanced...Suppose then, that A is both true and false; then so is not-A. Hence A and not-A is true; and, of course, false, as are all contradictions...

Sorensen (2001, p.147) commenting on these views of Priest states, '...Priest seems as much a skeptic about the existence of contradiction as he seems a daringly open-minded believer in contradictions.' However, either and both ways, denying contradictions and/or embracing them, on Priest's account, it is clear that contradictions are allowed, just as is the case for a-rational/primary process mentation.

We have certainly not exhausted all the positions on vagueness in this brief review. In fact, in a later section in this chapter important views pertaining to metaphysical or ontic vagueness are taken up. First however, in the section immediately following, let us return to the psychoanalytic realm in order to discuss the constitution of *a-rational objects*, a topic whose great significance to ontic vagueness I will then endeavor to demonstrate.

A-rational objects

Elsewhere (Brakel 2003, 2009, chapters 3 and 4) I have held that:

1) Freud's secondary processes map well onto Kant's 12 necessary categories.[13]

2) In situations in which primary process/a-rational thinking predominates— in dreams, neurotic and psychotic symptoms, and in much mentation of very young children—the type of 'according-to-the-categories' synthesis necessary to constitute regular objects as the consensually agreed upon, determinate objects with which we are familiar (e.g., tables, stars, dogs)— does not obtain.

3) Instead, under primary process mentation, a-rational *objects* are constituted by an *associationist* principle of combination, even though Kant held that from an 'objective viewpoint' an associationist principle puts representations together '… in any order…[which] would not lead to any determinate connection of them, but only to accidental collocations' (Kant 1791, A121, p.141).

With Kant's view of the 'objective' object in mind, I have continued to assert that nevertheless:

4) This primary process/a-rational type of associative combination principle was necessary and even prior to synthesis by the categories, if Kant was correct that synthesis by the categories is a combinatory principle in which a determinate organization puts them together as '…they are combined in the object, no matter what the state of the subject might be'

---

[13] Here is Kant's (1781/1787 [1965] A80/B106, p.113) table of categories. He arranges them into four groups, each with three categories. I—*Of Quantity*: Unity, Plurality, Totality; II—*Of Quality*: Reality, Negation, Limitation; III—*Of Relation*: Of Inherence and Subsistence, Of Causality and Dependence (cause and effect), Of Community (reciprocity between agent and patient); IV—*Of Modality*: Possibility–Impossibility, Existence– Nonexistence, and Necessity–Contingency.

In this chapter, in addition to page references for Kant's *Critique of Pure Reason*, there is either an A or a B followed by a number denoting the passage. A refers to the first (1781) edition and B to the second (1787) edition.

(Kant 1797, B142, p.159). For in my reading of this passage Kant implies 'that subjects cannot bind things together as they are combined in the object without having *contrastive* ground in an earlier and subjective putting together of these representations' (Brakel 2009, pp.48–49).

Let us have a look at some sample a-rational *objects* and see how they are constituted and constructed. A striking example comes from the psychotic patient discussed above, Mrs. M. Mrs. M was clearly hallucinating and acting on a delusion in which she associated her current tumor pain with the past pain of childbirth. This association lead to a conflation which was manifest as she experienced herself to be 'delivering' the a-rational condensed *object*, consisting of the hard plastic head and shoulders shaped bottle of 'Head and Shoulders' brand shampoo and the heads and shoulders of her newborns.

Other examples can be seen when children or animals do not divide up the world as we do. Owners taking their puppies to dog school are instructed that for dogs a person with a hat is experienced as a human being different from that same person without a hat; and likewise for people with or without backpacks, crutches, etc. My friend J, when swimming with her dog in murky water, found that the dog seemed to regard J's legs as not part of J. Unable to see the point of attachment, the dog began to attack J's legs. Human examples are plentiful too. Things that adults regard as separate, children can view as joined. For example, a child seeing a particular chair always tucked under a table might experience the whole thing as one object. Similarly for a fire and fireplace. Stars in the sky might be seen as a two-dimensional visual object, with the stars not considered separately.

Two things are clear in these examples. 1) The associationist combinatory law could not be what Kant sought as the binding principle in constituting 'objective' singularly determinate objects; and 2) it could not serve specifically owing to its primary process/a-rational qualities. Kitcher (1990, p.79) puts Kant's view thus: 'The law of association…links cognitive states related by spatiotemporal contiguity…[and] spatiotemporal contiguity is too promiscuous.' Indeed, object construction based on representations combined by association—without the constraints of the rational/secondary process/Kantian category-mediated constitutive process—must result in unwieldy, funny, not-readily-describable *objects*.

Notice that the discussion of a-rational objects in this section pertains to *our* epistemology; our constituting of objects from various representations. I have not addressed the relation between our construction of such objects and what is out there in the world getting represented by us. Kant's position, that we can only know how we know, and not what is out there in itself, must be kept in mind. However, to the extent that we have added to our knowledge of how we know—we now know that we constitute a-rational *objects* as well ordinary ones—intriguing questions about the ontology of both ordinary and unusual objects can be raised.

Similarly, the next section presents views on whether or not the world is vague versus vagueness existing just in our concepts. In both cases while the ontological questions are not the main focus of this chapter, they provide a fascinating side issue related to the matter that is our main concern—the emergence of a-rationality in various accounts of vagueness. We now turn our attention to views of ontic vagueness in particular.

Ontic vagueness

As in the earlier section describing views on vagueness, our interest here focuses on whether or not, on various accounts of vagueness (and the implications thereof), a-rationality emerges. This section specifically addresses this question with respect to diverse philosophical positions on vagueness in the world (ontic vagueness) versus vagueness only in our languages and concepts (semantic vagueness).

Views on vagueness in the world

Vagueness in the world: Not applicable

Bertrand Russell's (1923/1997) classic article 'Vagueness' takes the position that the very idea of vagueness (or preciseness) is not applicable outside of our representational systems: 'Vagueness and precision alike are characteristics that can only belong to a representation, of which language is an example. They have to do with the relation between a representation and that which it represents. Apart from representation...there can be no such thing as vagueness or precision; things are what they are, and there is an end to it' (p.62). He argues further that vagueness is also not in the knowing (which is an occurrence, neither vague nor precise) nor in what is known (from the world), but is strictly '...a characteristic of ...[the] relation [of the knowing] to that which is known...' (p.62).

A-rational analog   Unique among the positions on the ontology of vagueness to be explored in this section, Russell's view that vagueness is a function of the imperfect match between our representations and that which they represent and has no further applicability in the world does not admit of any obvious a-rational analog.

Vagueness in the world: No

The philosophers in this group, although largely in agreement with Russell, take a harder line on vagueness in the world. Michael Dummett (1995, pp.209–210), e.g., asserts: 'Vagueness is not a property of objects, in particular not of physical objects…There can be objects whose boundaries are vague: questions of the form "Are we in the Midlands/Gobi Desert yet?" may not always have a definite answer, and it is obscure what is and is not part of a person's body.[14] But this just means that predicates of the form "is in/on/a part of x" are sometimes vague…' Here is an example from RM Sainsbury (1989, p.101) demonstrating this point: '…it is one thing to say that it is vague whether such-and-such is a part of Snowdon,[15] and another to say that Snowdon is such that it is vague whether it has such-and-such a part. The latter forces upon one the view that Snowdon is a vague object, whereas the former is consistent with Snowdon being sharp and only "Snowdon" vague.'

Among the most widely cited arguments for vagueness existing in our concepts, but not in the world, is the following from Gareth Evans (1978/1997, p.317). He intends to demonstrate that since identity cannot be indeterminate, vague objects cannot exist, given that they would have indeterminate identity relations. He begins by assuming that which he wants to disprove, 1) that vagueness in the world exists, and 2) that owing to this vagueness identity statements between fuzzy-boundaried-vague objects would have indeterminate truth values.

1. It is indeterminate whether $a = b$.
2. Then b can be described as having a property whereby it is of indeterminate truth value as to whether $b = a$.
3. However, for a, since $a = a$ definitely, it is not the case that a has a property whereby it is of indeterminate truth value as to whether $a = a$.
4. Then a cannot be described as having a property whereby it is of indeterminate truth value as to whether it is identical to a.
5. Hence, since b has a property that a does not, it is not the case $a = b$. (This from 2, 4, and Leibnitz's Law.)
6. Determinately then it is not the case that $a = b$.[16]

A-rational analog   This view that vagueness is a function of our concepts and language, but not a characteristic of the world, displays emergent a-rationality,

---

[14] Is the sandwich I ingested part of my body? Does it become so? When? Is it as I put it in my mouth? What about when it gets broken up into proteins, sugars, and starches through the enzymatic activity in my digestive system? Or is it only part of my body when these nutrients are supplied to my bloodstream?

[15] Snowdon is the highest mountain in Wales.

[16] Note that this 'simple' proof has generated much discussion, particularly about Evans' true intent. An interesting article on that topic is that by David Lewis (1988/1997, pp.128–130) titled, 'Vague identity: Evans misunderstood.'

but in a subtle manner. While this account spares the *world* all of the difficulties associated with non-bivalent logics, it is our *concepts* that thereby cannot avoid inheriting the same difficulties with the law of excluded middle and in tolerating contradictions as was discussed above in the section on many-valued logics, etc.

Vagueness in the world: Maybe

Sainsbury (1987, pp.48–49) questions the conclusion of Evans' argument above. He disagrees that arguments demonstrating that identity is not vague can establish that vague objects (putatively because their identity relations would be necessarily be vague) cannot exist. He offers an argument for definite identity relations between vague objects:

1. If b is a, then b is definitely a; if b is not a, then b is definitely not a.
2. Suppose b is a.
3. Since for any object x, x is definitely x, for a, 'is definitely a' is true of a.
4. Since b is a, anything true of a, is true of b.
5. a 'is definitely a' is true of a; so 'is definitely a' is true of b.
6. Hence b is definitely a.

Sainsbury then makes his case, asserting that nothing in this argument precludes the possibility that two vague objects could be identical with one another since nothing precludes that the a and b in this argument could refer to vague objects.

Sainsbury (1990/1997) also proposed that vague concepts are better understood as concepts without boundaries instead of those that admit of borderline cases. 'A vague concept is boundaryless in that no boundary marks the things which fall under it from the things which do not, and no boundary marks the things which definitely fall under it from those which do not definitely do so; and so on' (p.257). These sorts of concepts classify not in terms of classical definitional criteria but '…like magnetic poles exerting various degrees of influence: some objects cluster firmly to one pole, some to another, and some, though sensitive to the forces, join no cluster' (p.258). Claiming that almost all concepts lack boundaries (p.252), Sainsbury notes that the use of paradigms, prototypes, and family resemblances (pp.258, 262–264) better determine the extensions of these concepts and categories.

A-rational analog Sainsbury does not discuss the nature of vague objects whose existence he argues for so ably in his 1987 proof. Thus, it cannot be ascertained whether or not on his view these vague objects would resemble a-rational objects. As for the type of concepts and categories he takes up in the 1990/1997 article, these show the 'usual' a-rationality in that there is no clear true or false as to whether various members belong. There is also something new. For Sainsbury, family resemblance and prototype categorizations play a central role in concept formation, just as they do in a-rational categorizations—in both the most significant similarity relations are predicated on associations between elements, some of which are small and inessential.

Vagueness in the world: Yes, but...

Mark Colyvan (2001) takes issue with Russell's (1923) conclusion that vagueness, although ineliminable in our representations, is not applicable to the world. Colyvan states that Russell's view can only hold if we 'have no reason to believe that the world is as our language says' (p.87). Then, following a version of Quine and Putnam's Indispensibility Argument, Colyvan contends:

> If vagueness is not eliminable from our language and if our best scientific theories are committed to vague objects, it would seem no fallacy to attribute vagueness to the world. Indeed naturalistic philosophers must take their guidance on such matters from our best scientific theories. If those theories require ambiguous or vague terms…a positive argument for the existence of such objects begins to emerge (p.91).

He proceeds with the argument in three steps:

1. We should have ontological commitment to entities referred to by terms indispensable to best scientific theories.
2. Terms such as 'species' and 'stars' are indispensable to our best scientific theories. In addition, these terms are vague; vague properties and compositional vagueness are attributed to them.
3. Therefore, we should have ontological commitment to vague objects.

However, note that, even though Colyvan has argued for the existence of vague objects, his account belongs in the 'yes, but…' group with respect to vagueness in the world. This is because his argument for vagueness in the world has nothing to do with the world as it is. Rather his pro vague-object view is entirely predicated on maintaining belief in the consistency and coherence of our own concepts and representational systems. Colyvan, in other words, answers the metaphysical question about vague objects in the world in terms of ontological commitments which really reduce to strictly epistemological commitments—commitments to our own epistemic vehicles, those concepts and representations of ours constituting our best scientific theories.

A-rational analog   Colyvan accepts vague objects ontologically. He does so as he presumes our best science, based on our 'best' (i.e., rational/secondary process) epistemological capacities, yields the best representations for approximating the world as it is. Would Colyvan accept the case I have advanced elsewhere (see Brakel 2002, 2009) for a-rational representations?

If so, would he be obliged to add a-rational *objects* to those to which he has ontological commitments?

Vagueness in the world: Yes

There are several different accounts that suggest there is indeed vagueness in the world. I discuss four of them.

1) Michael Tye (1990, 1994/1997) believes that there are vague objects, and that '…the world is, in certain respects, intrinsically, robustly vague…' (1994/1997, p.293). Among vague objects, Tye includes entities such as Mount Everest, a mountain for which there is no clear dividing line between the matter composing it and matter of which it is not composed (1990, p.535), abstract objects such as the set of tall men, and some properties or concepts such as baldness (1990, p.536). For Tye, vague objects are not simply semantically vague (1990, pp.539–540),[17] and they do not imply that the identity relation is indeterminate (1990, p.538). He finds all the major views propounding precise-world alternatives to vague objects implausible. These include the claim of those holding the epistemic view, that there are sharp boundaries (1990, pp.542–543); Peter Unger's (1979a, 1979b) claim that the world is precise, but ordinary (vague) objects do not exist (Tye 1990, p.543);[18] and supervaluationism, whereby countenancing vague objects can be avoided by the process of precisification—a process of sharpening the meaning of a sentence or term, P, such that P is true iff (if and only if) it is true under all (eligible) ways of making P completely precise (1990, pp.540–541). Regarding the last view, Tye (1990, p.541) argues that supervaluationism actually implies the existence of vague objects, as the sharpening 'seems to require that there be something…which is capable of being made precise. But nothing that is already precise can be made precise. So again it appears that vague objects…are needed.'

2) SC Wheeler's (1975) work on vagueness appears almost the obverse of Russell's, in that Wheeler suggests that when vagueness is present, it is not the concept that is vague, but the world. Using the concept 'tall men' as an example, Wheeler (1975, p.377) asserts that, 'we are sure that it has *no* referent when we are sure that whether an object is in the extension of its referent is not a matter of fact.' In cases like this, '…our confidence that there is no fact of the matter [determining the extension] amounts to confidence that

---

[17] In fact, Keefe and Smith (1997, p.49) state that, for Tye (1994/1997), recognition of the ontologic vagueness in vague sets is important in understanding linguistic vagueness.

[18] Unger's position is taken up at length below in the next subsection.

tall men are not a kind, that this predicate does not refer.' Note however, that whereas other philosophers would take this to indicate *semantic vagueness*, i.e., that the vagueness is in our concept 'tall men,' Wheeler contends that such a referent-less concept, a concept in which 'no real kind in the world to which "tall man" denotes' (p.379)...is the very essence of *ontological vagueness*' (p.370) [my emphasis]. Ontic vagueness, then, as he construes it, certainly exists for Wheeler. In fact he states, '...there is nothing puzzling about ontological vagueness beyond puzzlements about non-referring singular terms' (p.379). Thus for Wheeler vagueness, as is indicated by the imperfect matches between our representations of the world and the world, comes from the world and not our concepts and our semantics.

3) Most of the time, when philosophers examine the possibility of vagueness in the world they consider vague objects. Terence Parsons and Peter Woodruff (1995/1997, p.322) point out that there are other (better) possibilities for genuine indeterminacy in the world: 'The world consists of some objects and some properties[19] and relations, with the objects possessing (or not possessing) properties and standing in (or not standing in) relations. Call these possessings and standings-in *states of affairs*.' They continue, 'Then the world determines that certain of them hold, and that certain of them do not hold, but leaves the rest undetermined' (p.322). For Parsons and Woodruff, vagueness in the world—where there are states of affairs in which it is undetermined (neither true nor false) whether certain objects possess certain properties—is more properly understood in terms of the indeterminacy of the state of affairs, rather than to 'blame' indeterminacy, with more specificity than is warranted, on either vague objects or vague properties (pp.322–323).

An example of the Parsons and Woodruff view on vague states of affairs comes from another of Parsons' (1987, p.4) articles. He presents the following situation: One day you are driving and swerve to avoid a pile of trash at a particular point on a particular road. Then, the next day, as you drive by that same spot, you note a pile of trash at roadside. Parsons claims that there is a unique referent both for 'the pile of trash you swerved around' and 'the pile of trash that was by the roadside the next day'; but that 'there is no answer to the question whether the two piles are the same...because of a genuine vagueness in the [state of affairs of the] world, and not just because of a vagueness in our language' (p.4).

---

[19] Properties are to be understood as 'the worldly counterparts of predicates' (Keefe and Smith 1997, p.50).

4) JA Burgess (1990) takes up the question of vagueness in the world again in terms of the vagueness of objects rather than states of affairs. He observes that many physical things seem to have fuzzy/vague spatial, and/or temporal boundaries—is some tree on the hill or is it more properly considered on the plane surrounding the hill; just when does an human embryo become a human being (p.265), or a boy a man? In light of this, since for Burgess there *are* hills and humans, we are committed to the view that there are fuzzy things: '...almost all the macroscopic physical objects we talk about are fuzzy in this sense' (p.265). With his position so stated, Burgess (p.279) next describes a view with which he sharply disagrees, one in which the spatio-temporal vagueness of all of our usual objects is but a 'superficial phenomenon of only slight metaphysical import...[because] [s]uch vagueness, although undeniably *in* the world, is not *due* to the world...Rather, it is due to (deficiencies in) the language employed to describe the world.' Burgess then continues with the ontologic consequences of this position: 'If we wish to maintain that the sense in which the world is precise is really a "deep" sense, then we shall be committed to the view that, in the "deep" sense, hills, humans, tables and other vague objects do not exist[20]...at least that there are no hills in any metaphysically significant sense' (p.282). Claiming that vague objects like hills and tables are just the sorts of entities that are central both in scientific realism—they are the concepts and theories that constitute our best science[21]—and in common sense, Burgess (p.283) concludes, 'I prefer to cleave to the common–sense view that all physical objects are genuinely and wholly concrete, whether or not their boundaries are precise.' In other words, hills, humans, tables exist; they are deeply vague; and he adds (p.284) that it is the case that 'Precise objects, if there are any, then emerge as limiting cases....' Finally, '...hills and other vague objects are there independently of us; indeed they *were there* independently of us *millennia ago*. What is determined (in part) by us is which vague objects we refer to and think about' (p.284).

---

[20] Unger (1979a, 1979b), as Burgess is well aware, does take this position. Burgess refers to Unger's 1979a work in the notes section of the article under discussion. I take up Unger's position in the next section.

[21] In this way Burgess' view is similar to Colyvan's (see above), but he takes it one step further and in a transcendental direction: '...even if we were to accept the view that vague boundedness is an artifact of certain [of our] perceptual processes, since the scientific realist will regard such [perceptual] processes as "physical", I can see no reason to regard such artifacts as any less real than fundamental particles' (1990, p.284).

A-rational analog   Although not what this group of philosophers just discussed had in mind, the very consideration of ontic vagueness opens the possibility for the existence of a-rationally mediated *objects*—i.e., objects
different from the familiar, rationally-constituted objects of our ordinary
experience. These four philosophers did however allow ontic vagueness, and
no different than the other groups discussed so far, each of the accounts
described can readily be seen as analogous to an aspect of a-rational mentation. With respect to concept extensions of vague objects, for instance, there
can be no exclusive 'true or false' assignments in the ordinary mutually exclusive manner of everyday logic. This is because, on each of these views, there are
no facts of the matter about such concept extensions. In addition, this is the
case when the 'blame' is given to metaphysical vagueness, including vague
objects or states-of-affairs, no less than when vagueness is attributed to our
epistemological concepts, categories, or language.

Perhaps most importantly for the current project, the philosophers
affirming metaphysical vagueness lead directly to a diverse collection of
philosophers who radically oppose this view. For this latter group, whose
views are described below, the world is not vague. However, these philosophers are markedly different from those discussed above in the 'Vagueness
in the world: no' category. Each of the following philosophers, in order to
avoid vagueness in the world, posits non-vague worlds that are anything but
ordinary; worlds potentially having qualities quite suggestive of a-rationality.

World(s) without vagueness (but not without a-rationality)

The David Lewis account

For David Lewis (1986), vagueness is just in our thoughts and language.
However, the non-vague world to which he alludes looks quite unusual to the
uninitiated. Lewis starts out with a rather typical position: 'The reason it's
vague where the outback begins is not that there's this thing, the outback, with
imprecise borders; rather there are many things, with different borders, and
nobody has been fool enough to try to enforce a choice of one of them as the
official referent of the word "outback"'(p.212). However, as he elaborates his
metaphysics, a more interesting view emerges. He observes that there are
favored ways that we carve up the world, which provide restrictions on what
counts for us as constituting real-world objects. Pointing to our preferred, but
obviously limited categories in combining elements to constitute these real-
world objects, he says: 'Speaking restrictedly, of course we can have our intuitively motivated restrictions on composition. But not because composition
ever fails to take place; rather because we sometimes ignore some of all the

things there really are' (p.213). Lewis continues, 'We have no name for the mereological[22] sum of my left shoe plus the Moon plus the sum of all Her Majesty's ear-rings…we seldom admit it to our domains of restricted quantification. It is very sensible to ignore such a thing in our everyday thought and language. But ignoring it won't make it go away' (p.213). Thus, for Lewis, conglomerated objects, such as the strange assemblage he described above, not only exist but they are not vague. On Lewis' view vagueness is just in our categories and concepts and the objects we regard as falling under them.

A-rational analog   More than providing material suggestive of an a-rational analog, David Lewis's metaphysics allows one to grant all sorts of a-rational *objects* at least the same ontological status as our preferred, restricted, 'objective,' rationally based, everyday 'real world' objects. My psychotic patient's combination *object* consisting of the 'Head and Shoulders' shampoo bottle and the heads and shoulders of her newborns is as ontologically real as that bottle of 'Head and Shoulders' shampoo and the soapy liquid inside it. Similarly, the pain of childbirth from decades earlier merged with the pain of a current gynecological tumor is as ontologically real as any more familiar combination, say the tumor pain combined with other signs and symptoms of the gynecological malignancy. Further, categories like those formed by the neurotic patient with premature ejaculation and an elevator phobia, i.e., categories predicated a-rationally and centered on an (objectively) inessential feature—openings with jagged edges or surrounded with powerful mechanisms that could damage a person or one of his members—can be seen to have the same status as our usual restricted everyday categories, those formed rationally by sharing an essential feature, such as the feature elevators share with escalators.

Our rationally mediated objects are favored as objects, not because we are carving nature at its joints, but because of our human cognitive capacities and motivations. We see a chair as a discrete object, not a chair-plus-floor-plus-table leaf, because of our visual perceptual system (color receptors, depth and edge detectors, etc.) and our motivations (we design a piece of furniture with the expectation that it will fit our functional needs given our anatomy and conventions). A-rationally based *objects* also derive from our human cognitive and motivational processes, but in a much more primary process and idiosyncratic way. Mrs. M desired to have no tumor at all. This strong motivation fueled the associative condensation of the shampoo bottle named 'Head and

---

[22] Mereology is the philosophical study of part-hood—the myriad relations of parts to parts within a whole, and the relation of parts to wholes.

Shoulders' with those same named body parts of her children as neonates—and this combination formed the a-rational *object*. Similarly, the elevator phobic's a-rational category of 'apertures dangerous to a man's members'—formed using associative links that connected one single inessential feature—was motivated by this patient's unconscious fear of mordant vaginas.

Now, on Lewis's account, both our familiar everyday rational objects and at least some of the unusual a-rational *objects* are vague. However, perhaps the a-rational unusual *objects* and a-rational categories, particularly their formation on the basis of motivated associations, can help us understand the creative mind of a philosopher such as Lewis, who can posit non-vague combination-type entities existing in a world that is not vague. The combination entity constituted by the sum of Lewis's left foot, the moon, and all of the Queens earrings appears to consist of 'randomly'[23] associated items. Given that Lewis contends that all manner of entities such as these do exist, and further claims that they will not go away even if most of us ignore them or never consider them; I propose that their existence could only be imagined by him via a-rational/primary process associative operations. In this case an aspect of our human cognitive capacities—the ability to produce a-rational associations of this sort—is put in the service of the creative endeavor of finding solutions to puzzling problems in ontic vagueness—a very human motivation.

Peter Unger's view

Peter Unger also advocates a world without vagueness. Unger's non-vague world is unusual too. In persuasive fashion, Unger (1979a, 1979b) argues that ordinary things—tables, chairs, stars, rocks, mountains, cats, dogs, persons, etc.—simply do not exist, common sense appearances to the contrary notwithstanding. His case is made using a few different types of sorites vagueness arguments. The first one (1979b, pp.120–121), 'the sorites of decomposition by minute removals' is set up by removing a single atom from some particular ordinary thing, a stone. If one atom is removed, it is still a stone, in fact still that stone. If two, the stone is still intact. However, iterated until '…there are no atoms in the situation…' (p.121), Unger wonders how can we still think that a stone is there. Yet, we must think that that stone is still there since each of these atoms is removed one at a time, and one atom cannot make any difference. Unger resolves this typical type of vagueness paradox in a very atypical

---

[23] Such associations only appear random. Humans are unable to associate randomly. One association necessarily connects in some respect to the next one. This is why people, on their own, cannot generate random numbers and need random number generator programs in order to approach true randomness.

way, concluding that, '...there are no stones and, by generalization, no other ordinary things' (p.121).

The sorites of slicing and grinding (p.132) and that of cutting and separating (p.137) are equally interesting. Suppose that a table is dismantled by one-fifth and then this table-fraction is separated from the original or even ground up. One could plausibly avoid vagueness and hold that the table still exists both as a table and even as that particular table, if after each removal it would be (in principle if not in fact) possible to reassemble it. However, Unger is not impressed with this move. Even if this view were coherent, he maintains there would be a profusion of ontological entities, 'For one will...suppose as well that every table that ever was still does exist and also, presumably, every mountain and every lake, every star and every planet' (p.139).

There is also the sorites of accumulation (pp.142–144), where starting with nothing and iteratively adding one atom at a time, one at first has nothing but eventually gets something, say a table—although, as is the case with all vague boundaries, the point at which that occurs is indeterminable. Accumulation sorites can also generate a more typical type of vagueness problem: What if one keeps adding atoms one-by-one to a table and at some point gets an unwieldy item as big as a house; it is vague as to when the table stopped being a table. In addition, as if these problems were not paradoxical enough, Unger (p.145) also combines his sorities of decomposition with that of accumulation, and describes stones shrinking into nothing, only to grow into feathers!

How can all of these contradictions and paradoxes, born of vagueness, be taken into account and accommodated in some way? Unger does not posit vagueness in the world; instead he asserts, 'The most rational way of responding to the contradictions...is to deny application for the ordinary concepts: the concepts of stones, tables, feathers and sousaphones. These concepts do not apply. We cannot say, then, "All feathers are stones"...[we can] say "There are no stones"' (pp.145–146).[24]

---

[24] Peter van Inwagen (1990) is in agreement with Unger concerning the non-existence of ordinary things—*except* that van Inwagen allows that 'material beings' exist. To the extent that van Inwagen (with Unger) denies that ordinary objects exist, he too avoids vagueness in the world. However, in positing material beings—composed of 'physical simples (p.72) caught up in the life (p.87) of beings/organisms' (pp. 90,145), van Inwagen does have to admit vagueness in the world, both in terms of existence and identity. Indeed, as van Iwagen himself recognizes, his vagueness problems for material beings are of several sorts. One is familiar: is this particular simple caught up in my life or is it not (analogous to the question of whether or not any particular molecule is part of Mt. Everest.) Another problem is that 'life' and 'beings/organisms' are obviously vague concepts. Is a virus alive, even though it is dependent on a living cell to replicate? What

A-rational analog   There are two different compelling connections between Unger's work and a-rationality. First, by attempting to eliminate ontic vagueness, a move plausibly motivated by a desire to make more precise and rational the objects and states of affairs in the world, Unger, too, utilizes examples that are quite like contents devised under the sway of a-rational mentation. He evokes disappearing and reappearing chairs, limitless numbers of tables that turn into items as big as houses or as small as stones, all of these 'immortal'; and feather-stones, as well as any and all combinations of various objects or parts. Second, Unger's very arguments allow a-rational *objects* and categories to exist no less and no more than our everyday rationally mediated objects and categories. Since on Unger's view stones, feathers, and stone-feathers all have the same ontological standing; so too do a-rational *objects* such as vagina dentate-elevators and shampoo bottle-neonates. For Unger all of these entities do not exist; and indeed they do not exist equally!

Mark Heller's ontology

Similar to Unger, Mark Heller (1990, p.68) claims that there are no ordinary things, including no people: '…Sorites arguments can…be understood as being relevant only to language and not to reality…the words "heap" and "stone" and "person" do not apply to anything because of their vagueness…There are no

---

constitutes a being? The politicized question regarding human beings is not even the most vexing, if one considers the problem of an amoeba dividing. When the mother cell divides into two daughters, how many beings are there, one, two, or three? When did the life of the mother cell stop since she never died? (See Chapter 4 of this volume for a much fuller discussion of these amoeba problems.) A third problem concerns the matter of the many. Van Inwagen (pp.214–217) sets it up as follows. If man M has a small part removed he is M minus P1 and he is still man M. Then what happens with him when an additional small part is removed and he is M minus P2, and so forth, with him arriving as M minus Pn after many iterations of small-part removal? Is he still M? Unger claims that in such cases there would either be a huge population of Ms or (preferable to Unger) no man M at all. Van Inwagen opts for a vague set where some group of Ms, and some group of M minus Pns together constitute man M. Finally van Inwagen, given his views on material beings, realizes he must endorse ontic vagueness both with respect to existence and identity. Using bricks to represent his 'simples,' van Inwagen sets up an example in which many bricks compose X. He then asks (p.230): 'Suppose we rearranged the bricks…would X still exist? Given that X still existed, would X still be a [or even the same] pile of bricks?' He concludes that it is indefinite on both scores, and that his views on material beings '… make it almost impossible…to deny that there is real vagueness in the world—that is vagueness that cannot be accounted for by the Linguistic Theory of Vagueness' (p.282).

Although his forced acceptance of vagueness in the world might suggest a précis of van Inwagen's views really belongs in the earlier subsection 'Vagueness in the world: Yes,' because of his denial of ordinary objects and what appears to be his uneasy acceptance of ontic vagueness, I felt reviewing his work in the current section is more proper.

people, but this is only because none of the many things there are can properly be called a person.' Heller boldly rejects the standard ontology, and then offers a non-vague ontology as a replacement: 'What really exist are four-dimensional hunks of matter: the material content of filled regions of spacetime' (p.69).

To understand his view, let us contrast it with our conventional attempts to have unified ordinary objects such as a table. Regarding a table as we usually do, Heller begins, '…we might say that a table has unity because it stands out from its surroundings.' 'But,' he continues, 'the paradox is applicable to tables because of the very fact that there is no clear line between the table and its surroundings, either along any of the spatial dimensions or the temporal dimension' (pp.49–50). Heller's position becomes even clearer with his description of the object 'Maryalice' (p.55): 'Maryalice is the object that exactly fills the region that we would ordinarily describe as including the front half of my car and all its contents from noon until two. Maryalice would be described as being part metal, part air, part human flesh, part gasoline, etc.' Continuing, Heller (p.55) then states that Maryalice, '…this oddly structured (to us) four-dimensional hunk…could not have had any other spatiotemporal shape (including internal structure) than the one it actually has.'[25]

A-rational analog   Heller's view, even more so than those of Lewis or Unger, reveals a-rationality in constructing his ontology of the material world. On his negative account, like that of Lewis and Unger, there is no vagueness in the world, and for Heller, as for Unger, avoiding ontic vagueness eliminates ordinary objects. However, then we get Heller's positive account of world ontology: An account that strikingly relies on a-rational associationist principles, particularly association by contiguity in time and space. Although the table may seem to stand out from its surroundings according to our ordinary rational conception, from Heller's four-dimensional space-time view—just as for certain for a-rational thinkers—the object in question is actually constituted by the table plus what is contiguous with it spatially and temporally. Thus the table, the floor it rests on, the floor's carpet covering, the items on the table's top, plus the empty area that pre-dated the table and the new piece of

---

[25] There are two main problems with Heller's program. First, he does not offer any principled guideline for determining what constitutes part-hood and parts with regard to his four-dimensional hunks. Second, Heller talks of the essential properties of these hunks based on *their* natures rather than our conventions (pp.142,154) [my emphasis]. However, although Heller can see some of our ordinary conventions, would it not be the case that his views are still constrained by his human (if unconventional) thinking? How can a human with a human mind and its constraints know the nature and essential properties of four-dimensional hunks of matter?

furniture that post-dates it—all constitute the object; an object that is both a four-dimensional Hellerian hunk of space-time matter and an a-rational *object*.

With Lewis and Unger, a-rational principles are as possible as ordinary rational ones in terms of the construction of objects. Combinations based on a-rational motivations can be as plausible (and as not-vague) as those mereological combinations we would never consider and/or we would ignore if we ever did. However, some such a-rational *objects* and categories are indeed as restricted as those constituting our ordinary objects and rational categories, and these are equally vague. For Heller, a-rational principles, particularly association by space and time contiguity, seem identical to those he singles out as the organizing principles used in combining and constituting objects in the ontology of his universe—objects that are non-vague four-dimensional material hunks in space-time.

Conclusions

After reviewing basic principles of a-rationality and some classic views on vagueness, I have shown that vagueness and a-rationality have important connections and similarities. One such likeness is the basic importance of similarity itself. The puzzles of vagueness are made obvious by the sorites paradox, which turns on the *similarities* between n and $n + 1$ and between some entity minus n and that same entity minus $n + 1$.

As for a-rationality, the principles organizing a-rational categories have much to do with different sorts of similarity relations. Driven by associative connections, and leading to displacements and condensations, similarity by contiguity of place or time, and similarity by small or inessential elements are the most prevalent similarity relations operative in a-rational mentation. These account for most a-rationally mediated concepts, categories, and objects, including those predicated on various types of family resemblances.

Equally interesting is the following connection. Much as the attempts of philosophers dealing with the puzzle of vagueness often yield higher order vagueness—vagueness 'infects' the very remedy; these same hyper-rational moves also reveal underlying a-rationality—a-rationality surfaces in the very attempts at rationality. For example, take those philosophers who use some form of many-valued logic to replace the usual bivalence/two-valued logic system. Here, when asserting that 'X is bald,' the statement cannot be evaluated as simply True or False. Instead a-rationality (or something resembling it) appears; True, False, *or* Undetermined are all allowable responses. In addition vagueness remains too, as there are now borderline undetermined cases, and, more important, still no sharp boundaries. It is just as hard to determine where the boundary is between someone who is clearly bald and someone borderline bald, as it is to decide what number of hairs gained moves someone from the bald to the not-bald group and then from being not-bald to the hairy category.

Likewise, a-rationality infuses almost any attempt to make more rational and precise the contradictions of sorites arguments. With many-valued logic solutions to sorites problems, just as with a-rational mentation, the laws of ordinary everyday logic are not in place; there is no law of excluded middle, statements about vague categories are not either just true or just false, nor are they mutually exclusively so.

Now the very idea of vagueness as something 'infecting' our concepts and/or the world is not shared by all who work in these areas. Some hold that vagueness is ubiquitous in our language and concepts, but not in the world; some hold that the ordinary world of tables and mountains is vague and robustly so; and some in both of these groups do not feel troubled. Russell has an elegant view, locating the vagueness in our representations, with the world being just as it is, neither vague nor precise, these concepts not even applicable. Others have different interactionalist views. For example, one holds that the fact that our vague concepts fail to refer determinately reflects ontic vagueness, while others, using the exact same examples, take such ambiguities of reference to demonstrate semantic vagueness. Another interactionalist, noting that our ordinary but vague concepts, e.g., 'cell' and 'star,' are not only of the world but contribute to our best scientific understanding of the world, suggests that we should accept ontic vagueness. These views are all moderate concerning vagueness.

By contrast a group of philosophers who claim that the world is not vague sets forth unusual and radical ontologies having much in common with what would constitute a-rationally based metaphysics. Peter Unger, although positing a world that is not ontologically vague, denies the existence of common, everyday objects, including himself and other beings. This gives a-rationally combined *objects* at least equal standing with those that are predicated on our ordinary everyday logical principles.

David Lewis, on the side of vagueness of our concepts rather than vagueness of the ordinary objects they name—e.g., he holds there is not one 'outback' but many things with many boundaries fitting that description—distinguishes between the objects we recognize, because they fit with our restricted preferences about which combinations we countenance as object-constituting, versus the objects resulting from the mereological sums we ignore. These latter exist nonetheless—objects such as the one comprising Lewis' shoe and the moon and some of the Queen's jewelry. On Lewis's account then, a-rational *objects* would have at least the same status as ordinary everyday rationally mediated ones, including in both cases their vagueness; and, perhaps some of the a-rational *objects* would not even be vague.

Interestingly too, the connections between a-rationality and Lewis's associatively based ontology can 1) lead us to appreciate his creativity in positing his non-vague world populated by unusual combinations, typically and rationally ignored; and 2) actually lend a certain sort of evidential weight in favor of the Lewis view. If our a-rationally mediated representations allow us to know a-rational *objects* as possible objects, the mereological combinations held by Lewis to exist also become part of an ontology within our reach epistemologically.

Finally Mark Heller's account of non-vague objects—his four-dimensional hunks of matter in space-time—is such that it constitutes what amounts to an a-rationally based metaphysics. Heller advocates that the objects that do exist without vagueness are predicated on the a-rational/primary process associative principles of association by contiguity of space and time.

***

This chapter has shown that on many and diverse sophisticated philosophical accounts of vagueness, when precision and rationality are sought, vagueness infuses and a-rationality emerges—in our epistemological and ontological views, no less, vagueness and a-rationality arise, and paradoxically so.

References

Brakel, LAW (2001). Phantasies, neurotic-beliefs, and beliefs-proper. *American Journal of Psychoanalysis*, **61**, 363–389.

Brakel, LAW (2002). Phantasy and wish: a proper function account of a-rational primary process mediated mentation. *Australasian Journal of Philosophy*, **80**, 1–16.

Brakel, LAW (2003). 'Unusual' human experiences: Kant, Freud and an associationist law. *Theoria et Historica Scientificarum*: Special issue on Unconscious Perception and Communication: Evolutionary, Cognitive and Psychoanalytic Perspectives, 7, 109–116.

Brakel, LAW (2009). *Philosophy, Psychoanalysis, and the A-Rational Mind*. Oxford, Oxford University Press.

Brakel, LAW and Shevrin, H (2003). Freud's dual process theory and the place of the a-rational. Continuing Commentary on Stanovich & West (2001). Individual differences in reasoning: implications for the rationality debate. *Behavioral and Brain Sciences*, **23**, 645–666, and **26**, 527–528.

Brenner, C (1955/1974). *An Elementary Textbook of Psychoanalysis*. Garden City, New York, Anchor Books.

Burgess, JA (1990). Vague objects and indefinite identity. *Philosophical Studies*, **59**, 263–287.

Colyvan, M (2001). Russel on metaphysical vagueness. *Principia*, **5**, 87–98.

Dummett, M (1995). Bivalence and vagueness. *Theoria*, **61**, 201–216.

Dummett, M (1975/1997). Wang's paradox. In R Keefe and P Smith, eds. *Vagueness: A Reader*, Chapter 8, 99–118, Cambridge, Mass, MIT Press.

Edgington, D (1992/1997). Vagueness by degrees. In R Keefe and P Smith, eds. *Vagueness: A Reader*, Chapter 6, 294–316, Cambridge, Mass, MIT Press.

Evans, G (1978/1997). Can there be vague objects? In R Keefe and P Smith, eds. *Vagueness: A Reader*. Chapter 17, p.317, Cambridge, Mass, MIT Press.

Fine, K (1975/1997). Vagueness, truth, and logic. In R Keefe and P Smith, eds. *Vagueness: A Reader*, Chapter 9, 119–150, Cambridge, Mass, MIT Press.

Freud, A (1936). *The Ego and the Mechanisms of Defense*. New York, 1966, International Universities Press.

Freud, S (1900). *The Interpretation of Dreams*. Standard Edition, Vol. 4 & 5. Trans. and ed. J. Strachey. London, 1953, Hogarth Press.

Heller, M (1990). *The Ontology of Physical Objects: Four Dimensional Hunks of Matter*. Cambridge, Cambridge University Press.

Kant, I (1781, 1787). *Critique of Pure Reason*. trans. Norman Kemp Smith. New York, 1965, St. Martin's Press.

Keefe, R and Smith, P (1997). *Vagueness: A Reader*. Cambridge, Mass, MIT Press.

Kitcher, P (1990). *Kant's Transcendental Psychology*. New York, Oxford University Press.

Lewis, D (1986). *On the Plurality of Worlds*. Oxford, Basil Blackwell.

Lewis, D (1988/1997). Vague identity: Evans misunderstood. In R Keefe and P Smith, eds. *Vagueness: A Reader*, Chapter18, 318–320, Cambridge, Mass, MIT Press.

Machina, K (1976/1997). Truth, belief, and vagueness. In R Keefe and P Smith, eds. *Vagueness: A Reader* Chapter 11, 174–203, Cambridge, Mass, MIT Press.

Mehlberg, H (1958/1997). Truth and vagueness. In R Keefe and P Smith, eds. *Vagueness: A Reader*, Chapter 6, 85–88, Cambridge, Mass, MIT Press.

Millikan, R (1993). Thoughts without laws. In *White Queen Psychology and Other Essays for Alice*, Chapter 3, 51–82, Cambridge, Mass, MIT Press.

Parsons, T (1987). Entities without identity. *Philosophical Perspectives*, 1, 1–19.

Parsons, T and Woodruff, P (1995/1997). Worldly indeterminacy of identity. In R. Keefe and P. Smith, eds. *Vagueness: A Reader*. Chapter19, 321–337, Cambridge, Mass, MIT Press.

Pessoa, F (1932/1991). Ah! um soneto. In *Obras Completas de Fernando Pessoa*, Volume 2. 291–292, Lisbon, Atica.

Priest, G (1985–1986). Contradiction, belief, and rationality, *Proceedings of the Aristotelian Society*, **86**, 96–116.

Quine, WV (1981). What price bivalence? *The Journal of Philosophy*, **78**, 90–95.

Russell, B (1923/1997). Vagueness. In R Keefe and P Smith, eds. *Vagueness: A Reader*, Chapter 3, 61–68, Cambridge, Mass, MIT Press.

Sainsbury, RM (1987). *Paradoxes*. Cambridge, Cambridge University Press.

Sainsbury, RM (1989). What is a vague object? *Analysis*, **49**, 99–103.

Sainsbury, RM (1990/1997). Concepts without boundaries. In R Keefe and P Smith, eds. *Vagueness: A Reader*, Chapter 13, 251–264, Cambridge, Mass, MIT Press.

Sorensen, R (1985). An argument for the vagueness of 'vague.' *Analysis*, **45**, 134–137.

Sorensen, R (2001) *Vagueness and Contradiction*. Oxford, Oxford University Press.

Tye, M (1990). Vague objects. *Mind*, **99**, 535–557.

Tye, M (1994/1997). Sorites paradox and the semantics of vagueness. In R Keefe and P Smith, eds. *Vagueness: A Reader*. Chapter 15, 281–293, Cambridge, Mass, MIT Press.

Unger, P (1979a). I do not exist. In GF Macdonald, ed. *Perception and Identity*. pp.235–251, London, Macmillan.

Unger, P (1979b). There are no ordinary things. *Synthese*, **41**, 117–154.

van Inwagen, P (1990). *Material Beings*. Ithaca, New York, Cornell University Press.

Wheeler, S (1975). Reference and vagueness. *Synthese*, **30**, 367–379.

Williamson, T (1994). *Vagueness*. London and New York, Routledge.

Part IV

Agency

Philosophy of action

Chapter 4

Agency—'me'-ness in action

Introduction

There is a remarkable similarity to be discovered between what is at stake in two very different domains: 1) In the struggles of psychoanalytic patients to fully appropriate their own self-motivated direction(s) in life, i.e., their own 'me'-ness or agency; and 2) in the answers to a vexing philosophical problem: When I care about my survival, when I want to survive; just what is it that constitutes the 'me' whose survival I so much want?

The plan of this chapter is to present this discovery in the following sequence:

First, I outline several examples of the sorts of difficulties almost every psychoanalytic patient has in the task of integrating diverse and sometimes conflicting motives toward establishing and securing a coherent sense of self, one marked by recognizing oneself as the prime mover of one's life. I suggest that these difficulties can be grouped into a type of problem, one that is best understood as a problem of agency, rather than other, more typical psychoanalytic formulations. Then, in the sections that follow, I discuss issues of self and agency in several nonclinical settings, including first-person agency in the dream state. These sections provide a bridge between the clinical realm and that of the philosophical dilemmas.

Next, I offer accounts of several philosophical views on the desire for self-survival, specifically focusing on various ideas arising in attempts to answer a central question: When I am concerned with my own survival, just what is it that constitutes *me*?

Then, in the penultimate section I propose that, in essence, it is one's agency that is at stake—not only in the conflicts of the psychoanalytic patients, but also in the philosophical problems regarding our survival. Next, I outline my own view of agency, very much in line with the idea that agency can solve these specific interdisciplinary puzzles.

However, this view of agency is not without some problems. In the final section, I examine some new and potentially difficult dilemmas that arise for my account of agency, and then attempt solutions.

Psychoanalytic (and other clinical) 'me'-ness struggles

As I contemplated which psychoanalytic examples would best illustrate 'me'-ness conflicts, it became increasingly clear that every patient whom I have ever treated could serve. Thus, for ease of presentation and to insure confidentiality, I have made amalgams. However, before I have us plunge into the deep complexities of the analytic situation, let us examine a simpler type of case with 'me'-related problems, namely people with akrasia.

Akrasia

Akrasia or weakness of will is manifest when a person decides that one of two available choices is the better one and therefore the one he/she *wants* to do; and yet he/she freely chooses the less good choice. So, e.g., Henry chooses to stop smoking and thereby to forgo cigarettes when they are offered to him. Despite this, when Susan offers him a cigarette he smokes. Many theorists have speculated on the problem of akrasia, and I too have had something to say about it (Brakel 2009, pp.150–151; 163–165); but for the present work I will just take up Harry Frankfurt's unusual view since it highlights a position on personhood relevant to the conflicts with 'me'-ness I later address.

Frankfurt (1971/1988, p.16) contends that having 'second-order volitions' are necessary for being a person insofar as persons will essentially *want* (in a second-order fashion) their actions to be predicated on one set of desires rather than another. Thus, in Henry's case, his desire to smoke is first order, while his desire to no longer want to smoke is a second-order volition. Put plainly, Henry wants the desire not to smoke to be his will. Now for Frankfurt (1971/1988, p.18), it is clear that if Henry acts in accord with his second-order volitions, i.e., with the desire he embraces, he will be acting freely as a person. But what if he is akratic and acts on his first-order desire? Here, Henry, at odds with his second-order volition and his will, although still a person, can no longer be, according to Frankfurt, thought to be acting freely. Instead Frankfurt suggests that he 'may meaningfully make the analytically puzzling statements that the force moving him to take the drug [in this case to smoke the cigarette]…is a force other than his own, and that it is not of his own free will but rather against his will that this force moves him to take it.'

Frankfurt (1976, p.240) finds something like this 'akratic passivity' in various other mental events too: 'Thus there are obsessional thoughts, whose provenances may be obscure and of which we cannot rid ourselves; thoughts that strike us out of the blue; and thoughts that run willy-nilly through our heads. The thoughts that beset us in these ways do not occur by our own active doing.'

Ronald de Sousa (1976, p.220) does not agree with Frankfurt on these matters, explaining that '...some mental contents are sometimes *felt* [my emphasis] to be "external" to our self [e.g.]: obsessive images....' In addition, Terence Penelhum much more vigorously contests Frankfurt's claim: 'To say that the desire [that one does not want to be governed by] is not one's own...is to say something obviously false. This obvious falsehood can be given the appearance of respectability with the aid of philosophical theories...' (quote taken from Frankfurt, 1976 p.241, who cites Penelhum, 1971, p.670). Frankfurt says of his critic: 'Penelhum maintains that the desire with which a person does not identify himself is "just as much a part of him as that which he does"' (1976 p.241, citing Penelhum 1971, p.672).[1]

I, like de Sousa and Penelhum, also take issue with Frankfurt's views; at least to the extent that they imply that only person-endorsed second-order volitional actions are agency-driven.[2] For me both the akratic's consciously preferred but deferred action (the non-smoking) and the akratic act (the smoking) are not only internal to the person, but are the outcome of agent-driven desires. In fact, on my account, the akratic act is desired more, if only unconsciously so, as is evidenced by its successful performance. This follows from my proposal that desire has a constitutive function—the willingness to act toward its own fulfillment. (See Brakel 2009, 135–165.) Thus if one has two opposing desires, the one on which one is most ready and willing to act, is the one that will take place (*ceteris paribus*).

This leads to another serious problem I have with the Frankfurt account of akrasia, in which passivity wins out over activity as the not-wanted desires are considered externally based rather than internally driven. His position allows no room for *unconscious* desires and *unconscious* agency. These are both central to any psychoanalytic view of akrasia, which would minimally maintain that 1) unconscious desires are fueling the not-wanted, but desired, akratic acts and 2) that the akratic acts are actively performed by agents—agents not conscious about the agential aspect of these undesired akratic desires.

---

[1] Note that I have used Frankfurt's quotation of Penelhum even though the wording in Penelhum's article is different. Because the gist is the same, I surmise that since Penelhum's article appears as part of the proceedings of a conference, Frankfurt is quoting from an earlier version of Penelhum's work.

[2] As long as Frankfurt's view would allow agency to those he considers non-freely acting persons (and to the 'non-person wantons' he later describes), I would take no particular issue with his definition of personhood. As will be made clear later in this chapter, agency on my account is not restricted to humans, much less to those humans achieving 'personhood.'

With these considerations, let us return now to Henry. Interestingly, we would likely find him eager to endorse Frankfurt's view to the effect that when Susan offered him a cigarette, he accepted it because he was overcome by an urge to smoke, passively giving in to it. Further Henry would probably be relieved to regard this urge as external to himself, his own desires, and his own agency. However in this, Henry, like most psychoanalytic patients, would be repressing, then displacing, and most importantly externalizing this unacceptable aspect of his own agent-driven agenda—a desire to smoke this cigarette now—onto something outside of himself.

With Henry's conflicts in mind, let us turn now to the psychoanalytic composite cases.

Psychoanalytic cases

Since I am making the claim that agency is central to almost every psychoanalytic patient, the first two cases presented are amalgams of several patients. This will increase the range of issues taken up (as well as protect privacy). I have also asserted that agency, rather than other psychoanalytic formulations, might better describe the trouble at the center of most psychoanalytic patients. Thus, the third case presented here is more detailed, as it is a re-evaluation of a previously published case, in which the patient's problems are newly considered in terms of agency conflicts.

Mrs. J

Mrs. J was a homemaker in her late 40s with a solid marriage and four children, two boys and two girls. Her home life was quite satisfying—her children were happy and productive, her husband devoted and successful, and her marriage solid, she and her husband enjoying their partnership in most every domain. All of this stood in sharp contrast to her work life. Mrs. J certainly had a more than adequate intellect and yet she never did very well at school, nor did she succeed in the various careers she attempted. She first trained as a social worker and then as a teacher, but despite receiving adequate reviews found that neither occupation suited her. When she started her analysis she was a not-very-happy bookstore employee. Since her family did not need her income, I inquired why she chose that sort of work. Her reply was quite revealing. She loved books; from an early age she had in fact desired to become a writer, and had even showed some talent. So now at least she could be near books.

As the analysis progressed Mrs. J joined various book groups. After a while we would both note that she made remarks with increasing frequency to the effect that she could probably write as well as some of the authors discussed, if only she would write. When I asked the obvious question as to why she did not try her hand at writing, Mrs. J replied that she actually had written quite a bit in her childhood, both formally, with teachers commenting that she had real talent, and informally, in journals for herself. However, she continued, as a teenager she decided that it was just easier not to write. She came to this decision when she was enrolled in a special summer writing course for promising teenagers, which she summarily dropped.

Mrs. J remembered that her parents did nothing toward facilitating an understanding of this quitting, this clear acting-out action. This, she noted, was in marked contrast to her own parenting. She (and her husband) regularly help their children whenever they want to stop participating in anything— especially something for which they show talent. Mrs. J speculated that her mother had been envious. Her mother had longed to be a writer too, but after submitting scores of manuscripts, all turned down, gave it up, became a librarian, and never wrote again. Mrs. J decided that her mother really wanted a similarly mediocre outcome for her daughter, despite her paradoxical and very intermittent claims that Mrs. J was such a good writer that she would no doubt write a bestseller some day. Mrs. J's father was a different story. He insisted she stay in the writing course. A man with little education, he nonetheless was outraged at her quitting, especially as he was footing the bill. Finding his attitude no more helpful than her mother's seeming indifference, Mrs. J felt that for him it was not an issue of whether or not she was involved in writing, it was rather that she should 'behave' and 'be good.' Mother, father, and daughter fought about the writing class. Mrs. J ended up hanging out with a group of 'druggy' friends during class time, and her parents gave up, feeling frustrated and defeated.

What was missing in this whole account, I pointed out to Mrs. J, was her own feeling about the writing class; did she like it, did she like writing? She could not remember! As this material emerged in her psychoanalysis, she began to write for the first time in a number of years. At first she did not tell me about it, and then she did. She decided to join a group for writers, one in which a sample short story had to be submitted to be admitted to the group. She was accepted. This was the beginning of Mrs. J's making a real change in her life with respect to writing. After almost two years of participation in this group, and after a considerable number of analytic hours spent on her ambivalence, she applied and was accepted to a prestigious MFA program in creative writing. The program was located at a distant university, but attendance requirements were minimal; she would have to be there for only a few weekends a year and the rest could be done online. She was ecstatic…at first. As the first semester wore on, Mrs. J turned her work in with more delay and greater anxiety.

Finally she stopped submitting her assignments altogether. Although she seemed to herself like one her own kids, who at age 8 had had a similar (but temporary) symptom, she could not get herself to do the work.

Initially she claimed she *could not* do the work; she felt her writing was not adequate, despite good reviews from the estimable staff whenever she did present work. Then she wondered if she even liked writing anyway. She was miserable. After several weeks of not writing, she began again to write. True, she did not turn in assignments; but she wrote.

Mrs. J's work symptom began to remit with these non-assignment writings. She established that 1) she wanted to write, independently of anyone telling her she must; and moreover 2) that she liked writing, as much as she liked almost anything. With this stronghold of her own agency finally in place—she was someone who wrote and liked writing—she did not retreat, and we began to construct what had gone wrong. As a child and teenager the many things she did well and liked were consigned to 'those things my parents want of me.' This category included 1) writing (albeit with ambivalence from her mother), but also 2) succeeding (at least moderately) in school, and finally 3) being a good (happy, popular) child, rather than a problem kid (hanging out with drug-takers, getting bad grades, being truant, etc.). Since her parents wanted her to do well in these ways, she acted in accord with an unconscious determination that she could not want any of those things and still be herself, a free agent. So, she claimed 1) it was easier not to write—especially since for Mrs. J, like her mother, the only real success would be something grandiose; 2) that she preferred doing not very well in school anyway; and 3) through no fault of her own she just was neither popular nor happy. Thus, at precisely those points where her own agency actually coincided with her parents' desires for her, Mrs. J, unconsciously displaced her own agent-driven desires onto them, not 'complying' with her parents' (ambivalently held) wishes; and, more importantly, refusing to fulfill her own agent-driven desires.

Following the considerable work in psychoanalysis recounted above, the test for Mrs. J and her agency was soon to come. Could she still want to write, like writing, and write, even for an assignment? Or, would she not work, (unconsciously) constructing harmful transferences, in which she displaced onto her analyst and professors the attitudes she experienced her parents to have held? In other words, could she maintain her own agent-derived desires even if others had similar goals?

Mr. D

Mr. D came to analysis for many reasons, primary among them, a very troubling symptom, suicidal thoughts that were both recurrent and persistent.

At age 35 he was a moderately successful lawyer in a group practice. He was married, with two boys, and among his chief complaints was his feeling of disconnection from his wife, an emergency room nurse, whom he experienced as quite demanding. On reflection, he realized he always felt an uncomfortable distance with his clients and colleagues too, most of whom he also regarded as expecting too much of him. Only his close and warm relationship with each of his sons gave him hope that he could be helped; that, and realizing that he was not so far gone as to actually contemplate acting on his suicidal thoughts; he understood that killing himself would permanently scar his children. Besides, his type of suicidal thoughts required no action anyway, he explained. His suicidal phantasies were very passive—he would be dead, that was all.

Mr. D described his parents as odd. They seemed to raise him and his older sister differently from how the other parents in their neighborhood (an affluent suburb of a major city) raised their children. Whereas other families did activities together, and were at least somewhat focused on the needs and interests of the children, Mr. D's parents seemed to him to be only interested in themselves, more specifically in his father. His father was an accountant, and extremely exacting, as every one of Mr. D's behaviors had to be accounted for. Emotions were not something that Mr. D's father 'got.' He appeared to have none himself and was quite critical of the rest of the family if ever they should laugh, and especially if they would cry. Mr. D in particular, a boy, was not supposed to cry. If he did, his father would openly degrade him. Mr. D's mother, a high school accounting teacher, was much more forgiving, but did not stand up to her husband for herself, much less for her children. To the very present, Mr. D could not name one thing that his mother liked; everything was filtered through his father/her husband. Despite this, he experienced his mother as demanding too. She wanted him to be a model child and he complied. She wanted good grades; he got them. She wanted him to be a boy scout; he was. She wanted him to play high school sports; he did. Then there were the things his mother did not want for him. She wanted him not to do drugs and alcohol; he did not. She wanted him not to date until college; he did not. Both parents wanted him to attend the same college as his sister, and since he really had no problems with that school, he did. Finally, his mother and father chose his career for him too. They wanted him to be a lawyer and so he was; but Mr. D had never any excitement in his career.

Regrettably, Mr. D admitted that he had never felt much excitement in his marriage either. His wife was the active one in their dating and all through the marriage. What felt to him like her inordinate demandingness, we discovered, turned out to be just regular spousal expectations. She wanted to have sex on a regular basis and have it be enjoyable for both of them; she wanted him to work and earn a good living; she wanted to work too; and she wanted to have a nice house, and some children.

Even with his two sons, with whom he did enjoy a close relationship, something of the same pattern existed. Mr. D felt constantly put upon by the desires of everyone, even his boys. We learned that a component of his suicidal ideation concerned a persistent fear that he could not measure up to everyone else's desires and demands. The feeling that he might prove inadequate was unbearable, and so Mr. D spent his time in equal parts withdrawing, or becoming angry, accusing, and self-righteous. He felt quite depressed. This was the pattern until at a particular point in the analytic work, we began to see something different in the character of his depression. Instead of being totally preoccupied with suicide, if he let himself think beyond the recurrent wishes to be dead (and the steps he needed to insure he would not kill himself), he began to become aware of very hostile and aggressive phantasies directed toward his loved ones and me. This surprised him at first.

The turning point in the analysis came in the transference. Always a considerate and even compliant patient, two years into the work Mr. D wanted to stop lying down on the analytic couch and have his sessions sitting up. I wanted to analyze his desire. He did not. Although he feared my scorn much as he would have his father's in a parallel situation, and despite the fact that he feared I would be outraged, he sat. Soon we came to realize the importance of this seemingly trivial positional change. Mr. D *wanted* something; and it was different from what I—with my understanding that analysis proceeds most readily with the patient reclining—wanted for him. As we noted this extraordinary event, we could begin to appreciate that Mr. D had unconsciously arranged his life, both as a child and as an adult, so as to experience himself as someone without desires; passive, but eagerly trying (although with unconscious, smoldering, self-righteous indignation) to fulfill what everyone else wanted. His rage was projected onto others, with Mr. D the picture of 'innocuous and pleasing' passivity. However, we now knew that the passivity was active and actively (albeit unconsciously) arranged;[3] it was the central expression of his agency—his willingness to act.

Understanding this helped Mr. D find or re-find some desires of his own. It was neither quick nor easy, but by repeatedly, in almost every situation, addressing the question, what does *he want*, he finally became aware of his own agency. This ushered in a new phase of his treatment; and more importantly his life—as he grappled with a life of desires, including wanting that which was

---

[3] Shevrin (2003, pp.15–16) reports a similar case of active agential passivity.

unacceptable, unobtainable, conflicted, and inconvenient, as well as that which was satisfying.

Dr. X

Dr. X, a child psychiatrist, whose case I have discussed before (Brakel 2004, pp.267–277) came into analysis with a senior male psychoanalyst when she was 38 years old. She had a variety of problems, but the one most relevant to the topic here did not emerge clearly for patient and analyst until well into the middle of the analysis. It concerned a strange work problem: although able to see her patients, review papers for journals, and critique them for colleagues, she was totally unable to initiate creative work on any of her several ongoing academic projects. The word 'initiate' is important because if some esteemed male figure, older colleague, supervisor, service chief, mentor, offered any sort of suggestion, Dr. X could work very well, at least for some limited period until the symptom would return again undiminished in intensity.

The work in her analysis was just the same. She seemed unable to work until her analyst (another esteemed older male) would make some sort of remark, at which point Dr. X could associate and put things together analytically. She and her analyst noted that his comments need not even be pertinent to the issue; all he needed to do was say *something* and for a while the symptom remitted. They termed the problem an 'ego constriction,' a term that had not been in the literature, but to both parties represented some sort of disturbance nosologically located somewhere between an ego inhibition and an ego restriction. Patients with ego inhibition, owing to internalized unconscious conflict, are unable to perform a task that is well within their capacities. In ego restriction, the patient turns away from the anxiety-provoking activity, decreasing his/her functional capacity, but just in that area (Brakel 2004, p.268).

Dr. X had grown up with a loving and warm, but somewhat incompetent and highly anxious mother from whom she had lifelong separation problems. This included a bout of chronic school phobia at age 6. Her father was domineering, psychologically powerful, successful, and although charming, especially to those outside of the family, he regularly degraded his wife. This resulted (with her mother's compliance) in Dr. X's father being regarded by everyone as the only authoritative and adequate adult. Dr. X identified with her father, in his strength, but unfortunately also in his degrading attitude toward Dr. X's mother. The punishment for Dr. X's hostile degrading of her mother was to become incompetent herself. However, to be incompetent afforded Dr. X the regressive pleasure of being with her mother, just as did her school-phobia symptom.

The ego-constriction symptom could be understood as follows. For Dr. X, success at her own creative work was equated with aggression toward her mother. This Dr. X could not tolerate for long. When Dr. X reverted to her paralyzed, non-initiating phase, she could be both *with* her incompetent mother, and *like* her incompetent mother, represented now by the helpless analyst in the maternal transference. Under these conditions no progress was being made; no one was going anywhere, certainly not Dr. X who was self-punishingly incompetent too; and certainly not the analyst or the analysis (Brakel 2004, p.268).

Despite this, things could shift, but only when certain rigid requirements were in place, namely when some important male figure expressed the sort of interest in Dr. X's projects that she could interpret as his saying: 'It's OK for you to work like me, and to be like me. I am your father and I give you the go ahead for this project. And by the way, I also sanction your degrading of your mother. You are not really doing these things at all anyway; you are still little and doing them at my behest, as my henchman.'(Paraphrase from Brakel 2004, pp.268, 273–274.) Then, she could work with enthusiasm and excitement; but only for a short time, until the cycle started up again.

When I originally examined the material from Dr. X's case, it occurred to me that 'ego constriction' was quite a felicitous term which could very well represent a distinct kind of problem, related to, but unlike the two more familiar symptoms—ego inhibition and ego restriction. I speculated that people with ego constrictions suffered from a problem structurally analogous to those with perversions since in both types of pathology rigid conditions must be met to obtain satisfaction—sexual gratification in the perversions and pleasure accompanying release of ego paralysis in cases of ego constrictions (Brakel 2004, pp. 268–269). Indeed this may be a useful diagnostic distinction. However, there is something both simpler and more far-reaching to learn from this case.

Dr. X's problem was essentially a problem of agency. Looking at the most superficial layer first, the adult Dr. X repeatedly attempted to escape the full wrath of her superego (conscience) by unconsciously externalizing her agent-driven desires for creative achievement onto the powerful males. She arranged to believe that her projects really belonged to the father figures. More crucially, the deeper original problem, the conflation of striving for her own success with dangerous unconscious hostile drives directed toward her mother, was agential in nature also. This owed to Dr. X's unconscious internalization of her father's agential aims (and his views), whole cloth without any modulation. For Dr. X it was as though the following slogan obtained without exception: 'Just as the competent one strives to create, the competent one must hostilely degrade' Thus, insofar as these two very different drives were amalgamated, inextricably linked, for both father and daughter, Dr. X's manifest separation problems with her mother could be understood as being fueled by a more serious failure to separate her agential aims from her father's; she had not yet developed an agential agenda of her own.

A note on the prevalence of 'me'-ness problems in psychoanalytic work

As I claimed earlier, almost any one of my psychoanalytic cases could serve to illustrate the sort of difficulties with 'me'-ness under discussion in this chapter. This, in conjunction with the typicality of the three reports above, suggests that it might be useful for psychoanalysts to pay more attention to issues of agency than we do. For example, I am aware that in re-examining the case of Dr. X, now in terms of her agential problems at the center, I have a fuller understanding, broader and deeper, both in terms of her history and current adult functioning than I did when I wrote the 2004 article. In that earlier publication I focused mainly on the various mechanisms Dr. X utilized—identification, displacement, externalization, and projection; writing as though this constituted some sort of explanation. However, as it turns out, reporting on those mechanisms, without positing some sort of organizational core, was far more descriptive than explanatory.[4] Indeed, we psychoanalysts often talk of identification, displacement, externalization, and projection; and we talk of them in relation to disguising and defending against drives, desires, and wishes. But what are the distorting defensive mechanisms, if not part of one's unconscious agency? And what are the drives, wishes, and desires themselves, if not the very motives for our agent-driven actions?

More will be said about the close relationship of action, drive, desire, and agency in later sections of this chapter. However, first, let us explore some non-clinical areas where other 'me-ness' phenomena arise.

'Me' in dreams, play, and other phenomena

As above, before we take on the more complicated situation of dreams, where there are many levels of first person goings-on, and often conflicting agential directions, let us begin with more straightforward examples, starting with cases useful to consider under the heading 'Extended "me".'

---

[4] The nature of various sorts of explanations will be taken up in Chapter 6, the final chapter of this book.

Extended 'me'

Physically extended 'me': Simple partial extensions and simple global projections

In baseball, when fielders are wearing gloves, the glove is an extension of the players' hands as they move to catch the ball. Likewise when playing any racquet sport, players move the racquet as extensions of their natural arms, directing the pieces of equipment as they would their body parts. Similarly, when surgeons use forceps, these are extensions of their fingers and thumbs, grasping the tissue just as would be the case with their natural prehensile and opposable digits. In all of these examples there is an artificial extension of a portion of a person's physical agency—a partially extended 'me.' As I have experienced all three of these examples (don't worry not as a surgeon, but as a medical student on surgical rotations), I can attest that in each of these examples the tool, racquet, or glove is manipulated quite unreflectively, as though the extension really were part of the physical self.

Less intuitively obvious, but interesting nonetheless are the cases in which one's agency gets globally projected. Take golfers who hit shots into the rough. As they look for their ball, each asks, 'where did I go; where am I?' If there are several balls in a similar location, each golfer will say (ungrammatically), 'that's me!' pointing (happily or unhappily) to his/her own ball. Unlike with checkers or chessmen, where someone will talk of 'my knight,' or 'my pieces,' the golf ball is thought of as a pure agential projection—'me' and globally so, albeit a very reductive version.

Psychologically extended 'me': Pretend play versus the virtual world of 'Second Life'[5]

Pretend play, in which children are quite aware that they are engaged in make-believe,[6] provides another area in which to explore the varieties of 'me'-ness. David Velleman (2008, pp. 409–410) describes pretend play as consisting '... partly of doing things in the real world and partly of fictionalizing about them...these two activities proceed in tandem: the players perform real actions and then decide how to represent them in fiction, or they make up fictions and then decide how to embody them in action.' What is the nature and status of the agential agendas of children initiating such play actions? First of all, it does

---

[5] I owe my understanding of the virtual world of 'Second Life' largely to David Velleman's (2008) article.

[6] This is to be contrasted with some types of phantasies in which the phantasizer is not aware of the distinction between inner wishful contents and outer reality. (See Brakel 2009, pp.105–134)

seem clear that both activities are agentially driven. Velleman (2008, p.410) bears this view out and adds something more: 'What a child chooses to do as a make-believe pirate is attributed both to the pirate, as his action within the fiction, and to the child, as his contribution to the game.'

What I take from this is that there are at least two agent-driven activities in pretend play. One is a direct expression of the child's intention in the real world, e.g., when a child says, 'This stick is my sword,' the child's intention is to brandish the stick as if it were a sword. The other agent-driven activity is indirect, as the child attributes feelings, beliefs, desires, and actions to the pirate. Are these attributed attitudes *simply* the child's own feelings, beliefs, and desires? I think not, and Velleman (2008, p.411) agrees: 'If a player imagines that "his" pirate is angry...[h]e certainly has not mistaken his own feelings for the pirate's.'

But how are these attributed attitudes and actions related to the child and his/her agency? I think that what we have here is a psychological analogue to the simple partial physical extensions described above. Thus, as the tennis racquet is felt naturally (and unreflectively) as part of the arm capable of striking and directing the ball, the child naturally extends aspects of his own attitudes such that they can fit the new pretend situations. The tennis player knows the real boundary between arm and racquet and does not confuse them. The child knows what his own anger feels like, and uses this to imagine what 'his pirate' would feel if he were an angry pirate; all of this without the child himself feeling angry at all.[7] In pretend play, aspects of a child's psychological 'me'-ness are, in this rather controlled fashion, partially extended to the attitudes and actions of the characters.

The virtual world of 'Second Life' is more complicated. Here adults in an online virtual environment select and manipulate human-like figures, 'avatars,' through the Second Life virtual world. Players, who often choose avatars physically different from themselves in terms of gender, race, body type, age, etc., have had no role in creating the virtual world. Once one has an avatar and can successfully move it, participants can, through the auspices of their avatars explore the virtual world; they also can desire and procure various material items from Second Life vendors; and even have their avatars fall in love. What is surprising is that unlike the situation with pretend play, in Second Life '... participants do not generally attribute attitudes to their avatars at all; they simply have thoughts and feelings about the world of the game, and they act on

---

[7] A child, of course, can feel angry and arrange to have the pretend characters angry as well. However, as the distinction between the child's feelings and those attributed to the characters becomes less distinct, the activity becomes less characteristic of pretend play.

that world through their avatars but under the motivational force of their own attitudes' (Velleman 2008, p.411–412). Thus when avatars 'fall in love' players describe themselves as in love! In short, a player in Second Life '…intends, not to make his avatar do things, but rather to do them *with* his avatar or to do them *as* his avatar, or…simply to do them' (Velleman, 2008, p.413).

More surprising still is that participants in Second Life report that they do not act with aspects of their own personality when engaged with their avatar in the virtual world. Instead, according to Velleman (p.415), '…they act in ways characteristic of the avatars, whose personalities are often very different from their own…'[8] Despite this, it is the player who constitutes the personality of the avatar. How can we understand the nature and status of a participant's agency in Second Life?

Velleman (2008, p.405) asserts that the selves created in such virtual worlds are composites of real minds and fictional bodies, acting in a fictional environment. This seems fine as far as it goes; the player agentially drives and directs the avatar. But what are we to make of the contrasts between players and their avatars? Some of the physical differences may not be that hard to figure out. If an older person selects a young avatar, a wish fulfilling phantasy of being young again is a pretty safe guess for his/her motivation in this case. If a physically disabled person has a robust avatar, again a straightforward wish-fulfilling phantasy of physical well-being is likely. But how can personality differences be understood? In the pretend-play case, the child's attitudes and actions are merely extended to the fictional characters. Not so here. One possibility is to view the personality, attitudes, and actions of the agent-driven avatar's behavior as illustrative of a psychologically extended but also *disguised* 'me'-ness, rather than as a simple psychological extension of the participant's 'me'-ness, as would be the case in pretend play. Take, for instance, a mild-mannered 35-year-old, white, male physician with gray hair and a full beard who selects a virtual life avatar who is 60 years old and Asian, an electric guitar player by profession, with no facial hair, false red dreads, and who behaves in a rowdy, bawdy, raucous way. Although we can know that the creation of this avatar is agency-driven, we cannot figure out just what combinations of desires, beliefs, and intentions—including extensions, disguises, and distortions—motivate this particular result.

---

[8] Writers of fiction often claim that the characters they create have a mind of their own and a life of their own. However, there is an essential difference. Fictional characters and the situation they find themselves in are both created by the same author. In Second Life the virtual world is as unknown and surprising to the human participants as it is to their avatars.

I will offer one final analogy. As we have established, the behavior in pretend play is agent-driven and derived from some psychological extension(s) of the player's 'me'-ness. In its relative straightforwardness, agency in pretend play resembles that in daydreams. Avatar behavior, on the other hand, while no less agent-driven is more complicated and derives from psychological disguises as well as extensions of the player's 'me'-ness.[9] The intricacies of the distorted disguises are such that the nature of agency involved in directing virtual world avatars more resembles the complex agential situation in dream states.

Thus, it is time to turn to the exploration of agency in dreams.

'Me' in dreams

When dealing with dreams, there are four levels of agency one must consider. Let us take Person Z, a patient in analysis as our exemplar dreamer, and let us begin with the most obvious level of agency: Z is an awake agent, both before and after sleep and dreams. Before he falls asleep we can guess that, at the least, he desires to have a good night's sleep. Maybe he is thinking about his plans for the next day, hoping things go well. When he wakes up, if he is like most analysands, he wants to remember his dream.

The next three levels of agency require that we review the process of dream formation as far as it is understood in psychoanalytic theory.[10] (See Freud 1900 for the full account; and Brakel 2009, pp.51–53 for a very abbreviated version.) The manifest dream content arises out of a complex operation that begins with an infantile wish that is stirred up by some current-day conflict. Often, both the infantile wish and its present day cover version are unconscious, having been rendered such insofar as they represent desires unacceptable to the mature person. Here is an example of how this can work. Z, whose childhood was marred by an older brother who often beat him up and attempted to degrade him, was yelled at yesterday by his boss. The boss, who happens to be older than Z, unfortunately uses his position to bully employees. As a child Z would sulk and storm, phantasize killing his brother while feeling helpless, especially as the brother seemed to be his mother's favorite. Regarding his boss, Z felt

---

[9] Disguises of one's agency are of course agentially-driven too.

[10] Although more is known about REM (rapid eye movement) sleep, both in terms of its causes and possible functional roles, the scientific status of dream content and formation is still mysterious and highly contested. Since views consistent with psychoanalytic theory cannot (so far) be ruled out, I will employ that theory here, particularly as the psychoanalytic explanations continue to provide more explanatory power than do any alternatives. (This was substantiated by Alan Eiser, a University of Michigan dream researcher, personal communication, 2009.)

furious for an hour but then forgot the incident. With this information we have enough to speculate as to the content of the infantile conflict and its present-day edition, both containing the second level of Z's agency: Z has an unconscious desire to kill the bully.

During Z's sleep that night a dream is formed. Here is its manifest content:

> I'm with my mother at a shooting range. She's using a big rifle to shoot at a target that mostly consists of a yellow bull's eye. Although her aim is terrible—her shots are never anywhere near the target—suddenly the target just disintegrates.

This manifest dream arises as a compromise between expressing and disguising the unconscious and unacceptable desire to murder. In addition, this very desire to both express and distort/disguise the composite unacceptable desire *is* Z's third level of agency.

The ambivalent desire to express and disguise can only be instantiated by employing what Freud termed the 'dream work,' non-conscious mechanisms that transform the latent content (wanting to kill the bully) into a manifest dream content that seems far more benign, if difficult to understand. The difficulty in understanding is because the resultant manifest dream, and the dream work mechanisms, all operate according to 'a-rational/primary process' principles.[11] These earlier modes of human mentation are different from the basically rational and logical 'secondary processes'; the 'primary processes' are neither rational nor logical. When primary process mentation obtains, the law of excluded middle does not hold, there are no negations, cause and effect is not in place, parts can stand for wholes, time passage is not recognized, and categorizations are made on the basis of insignificant features. The primary process dream work mechanisms include part-for-whole categorization, displacement and condensation (of contents), plastic representation, and secondary revision/secondary elaboration, this last giving the dream a façade of coherence, so that one is capable of remembering the dream and recounting it at all.

Returning now to Z's manifest dream, even without his associations (necessary for analyst and patient to adequately understand dreams) a lot of the dream work mechanisms are obvious. We can see plastic and part-for-whole representation in the bull's eye standing for the bully; and the yellowness of the bull's eye both for the boss's 'yelling' and for cowardice. Displacement is evident, in that his mother, not Z, is doing the shooting; and it is via condensation that bull's eye can represent both the new and old bullies. Further, causal

---

[11] See this volume, Chapter 3 for a review; and Brakel (2009) for a more complete account of the nature of the 'a-rational primary processes.'

relations do not hold as the target disintegrates. In addition, since Z did recall the dream and was able to report it, secondary revision/elaboration was present too. Third-level agential desires succeeded.

To get to the fourth level of agency, the 'me'-ness in the resultant manifest dream itself, Z's associations to the dream and its elements are needed. Here they are:

> My brother is her first child, so maybe that's why she preferred him. She'd never shoot him. She'd never even back me up when he came after me, yelling. Oh yeah like my boss yelling. Yellow, I feel I'm yellow in just plotting to kill him, and never really doing anything to him. Neither to my brother nor to my boss; I always back off and forget how angry I feel. I guess I'm afraid that if I know how mad I am and I try to even the score, it'll backfire, and I'll be the one to lose everything.

Different portions of this meaningful material would be relevant to Z at various points in his analysis. Early on, e.g., one might interpret that he fears disintegration if he so much as becomes aware of his hostile desires toward his brother and/or his boss. Later, the analyst might suggest that Z has a number of aggressive desires toward his brother, the bull's eye, exacerbating his feelings toward his boss—for instance, the analyst might interpret that Z wishes his brother were the 'yellow' cowardly one; and, moreover that his brother and boss ought to disintegrate, and become easy targets. However, the task in understanding Z as an analysand in the clinical situation—a task that certainly includes comprehending his most important agential desires—is different from the academic task at hand in elaborating instantiations of this patient's 'me'-ness in the manifest dream, the fourth level of agency in dreams.

Therefore, in order to uncover the fourth level of dream agency we need to find the driving force(s) behind the actions and behaviors of the various manifest dream character(s). First, we notice that in Z's dream his mother is obviously the active agent, while Z himself is just there. However, it seems evident that Z animates the manifest dream figure of his mother with his own agential agenda insofar as *she* has Z's conflicted motivations, both in trying to shoot her bully son (boss), and being too incompetent to do so. Thus we can say that in the manifest dream Z's first person agency is largely displaced onto his mother. In line with this displacement note that another agentially driven desire is expressed. Not only does Z wish to shoot his brother, he wishes his mother would wish to shoot him. Finally, there is another important representation of Z's agential 'me'-ness in the manifest dream, one without displacement, in which Z appears as himself: Z is alone with his mother, representing as fulfilled his agential desire that he be the first and only son.

Like the avatars in Second Life who have personalities, attitudes, and drives differing from those of their players, the persons appearing in manifest dreams can be other than the dreamer. Yet in both Second Life and in manifest dreams the agency, the very 'me'-ness of the dreamer and the player is always represented, albeit in uniquely transformed ways; disguising the agent's first person-ness via various primary process mechanisms. This similarity between Second Life avatar agency and the fourth level of dream agency is perhaps the most important. However, the first three levels also show parallels. For agency level one, the player wants to play and play with some coherence, just as the soon-to-be-dreamer wants to sleep and then remember coherent-enough dreams. In agency level two, for the players of Second Life just as for dreamers, there are unconscious desires, probably both infantile and current-day versions, which the player (as the dreamer) regards as unacceptable. At the third level of agency, players like dreamers have the unconscious motivation to distort and disguise these unacceptable attitudes; and they do so using unconscious primary process mechanisms, carrying out this unconscious agential directed act.

Having employed psychoanalytic theory to explore instantiations of 'me'-ness through one's agency in a variety of clinical and non-clinical situations and states—in akrasia, and psychoanalysis itself, in pretend play, virtual world games, and in the dream state—it is time to turn to a particular type of philosophical concern, one that I intend to show is deeply related to the above investigations. I characterize the philosophical problem with a single question: When I care about my survival, when I want to survive; just what is it that constitutes the 'me' whose survival I so much want?

Philosophical concerns about my survival: What constitutes 'me'?

The amoeba problem

As a young person, I was thrilled when I first learned in biology class about amoeba reproduction. It seemed to me that these single-celled organisms had found a way to resist inevitable mortality. An amoeba first reduplicated the material in its nucleus, and then divided, with each resultant cell having half of this doubled amount, i.e., the normal amoeba nucleus, and then both of them going on to live normal amoeba lives until it was time for them to reproduce.

I was thrilled anew to find that the amoeba situation provides a model for a set of very serious philosophical problems concerning 'me'-ness.[12] The first problem can be introduced with a seemingly simple question regarding the

---

[12] Philosophers including David Wiggins (1967), Derek Parfit (1984), Robert Nozick (1981), and Bernard Williams (1973) have all contributed to the literature on this matter.

amoeba(s) after reproduction: Suppose that I am the mother cell amoeba. Just what is my ontological status, once the two daughter cells are produced? True, I did not seem to die. But am I still alive, and if so what does that mean? Could I be alive *as* me and *as* my two daughter amoeba cells? An important issue arises here concerning numerical identity versus exact similarity. (See Penelhum 1955/1970, p.65; Prior 1965–66, pp.189–190; Williams 1956–57/1973, pp.9, 23–25; Nagel 1986, p.27; and Parfit 1984, pp.201–202.) Take some single count thing—an X, this particular X. This particular X can change over time and still be this particular X. But can this particular X still be this particular X if there are now two of them? The problem remains and actually intensifies if the two Xs are more like what had been the original particular X, than is that original X that has undergone changes over time. (In other words, there are two Xs at time $t + 1$ that are exactly similar to what the original X had been at time t, but the original X at time $t + 1$ is not exactly similar to what itself had been at time t.)

Clearly, there are serious 'me'-ness issues involved, and they are not restricted to amoebas, nor to children or academics imagining their deathless lives as amoebas. Theoretically, anyway, people could undergo a sort of fission too. There are also other thought-experiment fates that we humans could endure, all engineered by philosophers in order to better understand what constitutes the 'me'-ness with which we are each concerned when we desire our own survival. An elaboration of a number of these cases follows.

Human fission

There are several variations on the theme of human fission.[13] One version of the basic story is as follows: You are about to die of a cardiac arrest. Your brain, however, is in good shape and can be transplanted, and there are three possibilities. 1) Your brain is transplanted into a clone of you that had been prepared for this eventuality; 2) Your brain will be transplanted into a non-carbon-based replica of you, made ready as above; 3) Your brain will be transplanted into another person's body. The body is in good shape, as the person suffered a sudden but discrete brain death. Moreover, the body resembles yours. This third case can be made more interesting if the other person happens to be your identical twin!

Now for some variations: The first one concerns the opening setup. Now you have been about to die, but you do not. The surgeon still believes that soon you will likely have the predicted cardiac death, but can no longer be so sure.

---

[13] David Lewis (1976, pp.24–29), Parfit (1984, pp.261–266), Wiggins (1979), Williams (1960/1973), and Nozick (1981, Part I, Chapter 1) each discuss this topic, or matters closely related.

Since humans can thrive with only half of a brain, the surgeon removes for transplant only one-half of your brain, leaving the other half for you. Changes in the three possibilities follow from this: 1a) You and your clone are alive, each with half of your brain; 2a) You and your non-carbon replica are both functioning, each with half of your brain; 3a) You and the formerly brain-dead other, your identical twin, are both alive each with half of your brain.

The next variation continues from the above. Your heart does give out, and so the half-brain that had remained with you is now to be transplanted. Here are the various possible surgeries: 1b) Your half-brain is transplanted into another clone of you, identical to the first one. 2b) It is transplanted into another non-carbon replica of you, also identical to the first non-carbon replica of you. 2c) It is discovered you were actually not a twin but a triplet, and the third triplet has suffered the same fate as the second one, namely a sudden brain death. Now your half-brain is transplanted into the third triplet, so both of the two surviving triplets are alive and well, each with a fully functioning half of your brain.

Several pressing questions arise. Under which situations are you surviving *as* yourself? If your original body is dead, but your brain is functioning inside a clone, or a replica, are *you* surviving as you but in a new body? What about if your heart held out such that you were still alive with half of your brain, while the other half went to a clone, a replica, or a twin? Can they not be surviving *as* you, as long as *you* are still alive? But then what about when you die? *Now* are they *you*, when before they were not? Finally, the case most like that of amoeba fission: Your original body is gone, but two bodies, either clones, replicas, or two of your triplet sib-ship, each have half of your brain. Do you survive now *as two* of you? But then suppose then that one of the triplets dies shortly after the transplant? Does the fact that there is again only one change the *you*-status of the remaining triplet? What if the amoeba reproduction did not go correctly and the fission was asymmetrical such that when it was completed, there was one big cell and one smaller defective one that later died. Would the big cell be the mother amoeba surviving, rather than dividing, or would the big cell be the only surviving daughter cell?

For now, these questions will remain unanswered. We will return to them later. But first, let me present another thought experiment situation in which some clear-cut positions are taken.

Body/brain exchange: Am I my psychology? Am I my brain?

Bernard Williams (1970/1973) describes Person A and Person B undergoing what amounts to an exchange of brains, although one could consider the operation to be either a brain or total body transplant.[14] Before the operation A and B are both told that, after the exchange, one of them will experience extreme pain and the other will not have any pain and will in fact receive a great deal of money. They are each asked which body and which brain they would prefer to endure the pain and which they would choose to have the good fortune. Suppose that Person A opts for future pain in the A-Body which will then have the B-Brain; and Person B also opts for future pain in the A-Body which will then have the B-Brain. Given these choices, the surgeon will be able to satisfy both patients with their before-transplant wishes, and we can examine how each will fare.

Clearly, assuming that both Persons A and B would like the non-painful financial reward for themselves, we can see that the pre-exchange Person A locates his/her 'me'-ness in the brain, whereas the pre-exchange B has his/her 'me'-ness in the body. Which of these positions makes more sense? Which patient does better? Williams suggests that mostly it has been assumed that Person A's view, that my 'me'-ness is in my brain, is more rational (1970/1973, p.51); and indeed after the surgery the person with the B-Body, the A-Brain, a lot of new money, and no pain would agree. Even the post-surgical B-Brained/A-Bodied person, feeling pain and having no financial compensation, would admit to the mistake.

Williams, however, gives a stunning case example that strongly suggests the contrary (1970/1973, pp.51–52)—namely, that the brain as the center of my psychological 'me'-ness, at the end of the day, is not all there is to 'me.' I will abbreviate his argument and (unlike Williams himself) continue to use most aspects of the original thought experiment involving Person A and Person B and their body/brain exchange. I will, however, stipulate a few alterations.

Suppose now that I am Person A. The surgeon tells me a few things about the operation: 1) The brain exchange will be that of brain software, rather than hardware, such that all of my brain-mediated psychology will be transferred to B's brain hardware, and vice versa; and 2) that sometime in the very near future, in preparation for the body/brain-exchange procedures, my body will be in a lot of pain. It is true that at that time all of the contents of my brain will be on the way to being exchanged and transplanted into the hardware of Person B's brain (and body), just as Person B's brain contents will be on its way to my physical brain (and body), but this too will require some interventions. First, at just about the time the severe pain in my body will begin, my brain (the A-Brain) will begin to lose all of my memories; in fact as the pain in the A-Body

---

[14] Williams (1970/1973, p. 47) attributes this thought experiment to Sidney Shoemaker (1963) *Self-Knowledge and Self-Identity*, Cornell U Press, Ithaca NY, p.23.

will continue and probably increase, all of my brain's psychological connectedness to me will be halted. At this point, and until the (my?) A-Brain hardware
receives Person B's psychological software, it will in effect have no psychological contents at all. Should I (Person A) feel heartened by this?

Williams (1970/1973) says certainly not, as he likens this state to 'being
involved in an accident...as a result of which I wake up in a completely amne-
siac state and also in great pain' (p.52). The surgeon then describes the next
phase: my, or perhaps more accurately, 'the' now psychologically empty brain,
will be connected up with all of B's memories and B's other psychological content, as the pain in A's body will continue to intensify, reaching the level of
torture. Should I (Person A before the exchange operation) now feel relieved
that all of the pain the A-Body (a.k.a. my own body now) will experience and
endure will be grappled with by a brain that will at that time be psychologically
B's brain? Again, Williams (190/1973, p.52) says emphatically no: 'Fear, surely,
would be the proper reaction and not because one did not know what was
going to happen, but because in one vital respect...one did know what was
going to happen—torture which one can indeed expect to happen to [one's
body, i.e.,] *oneself* [my addition and my emphasis]...'

With this line of reasoning, based on a thought experiment demonstration,
Williams (1956–57/1973, p.1) makes good on his aim to '...try to show that
bodily identity is always a necessary condition of personal identity.' This is
an argument for physicalism, extending beyond brain physicalism, about
'me'-ness.

Thomas Nagel (1986, p.42) embraces physicalism too, but in a more specific
brain-based fashion. Arguing that although in thought experiments, such as
those above, one may be able to *imagine* that one is still oneself divorced from
one's brain, if one cannot really *be* oneself without one's brain, such imagining
will show one to have '...confused epistemologic with metaphysical possibility.' He continues, 'In trying to conceive of my survival after the destruction of
my brain, I will not succeed in referring to *myself* [my emphasis] in such a
situation if I am in fact my brain' (p.42). For Nagel, it is the case that he cannot
be Thomas Nagel without his brain. When he cares about his survival then, it
cannot be without his brain. '...if a physically distinct replica of me were produced who was psychologically continuous with me though my brain had been
destroyed, it would not be me and its survival would not be as good (for me)
as my survival.'

Nagel, here, is directing his arguments to the position of Derek Parfit, who
does hold that it is (or at least should be) psychological continuousness and
psychological connection that matter when we are concerned about our survival; this more than personal identity, including personal identity that is body

and/or brain based. I turn now to Parfit's interesting account, particularly a group of further illustrative thought experiments he constructed.

Teletransporting, physical and psychological spectra, and 'Relation R'

Derek Parfit (1984, pp.199–201) uses a science-fictional device, teletransportation, in order to engagingly elaborate his views on what constitutes personhood and what it is we do and *should* care about when we are interested in our own survival. In teletransportation, a person, let us call him D, presses a button to signal his readiness to begin the process and then after some time has elapsed is rendered unconscious. He next undergoes a procedure where his body, including his brain, is totally destroyed, but then body and brain are reconstituted on Mars. This takes place on a cell-by-cell basis, as the status of each cell is registered on Earth and then programmed into organic material available on Mars such that Mars-D is indistinguishable from Earth-D both physically and psychologically.[15] The Earth version of Person D never regains consciousness, while the Mars version experiences himself as D, physically and psychologically, with no doubts at all.

On Parfit's view, Person D should not have much trouble with this—Mars-D is a perfect physical replica of himself, and no less organic; moreover, Mars-D is totally psychologically connected and seamlessly psychologically continuous with Earth-D. In addition, to the extent that Person D embraces Parfit's position, namely that it is precisely the preservation of *Relation R*—consisting of psychological connection and continuity of his body and his brain's contents—that is essential to survival, Earth-D and Mars-D, either and both instantiations of Person D, have no trouble whatsoever with teletransportation and self-identity. In fact, D makes several round-trips in teletransporting. It is of note that, on Parfit's account, Relation R[16] is not only different from *personal*

---

[15] Parfit suggests a modified physicalist brain-based psychology here.

[16] Relation R for Parfit (1984, p.206) consists of psychological connectedness, 'the holding of particular direct psychological connections,' and psychological continuity, 'the holding of overlapping chains of strong connectedness.' Psychological connectedness can be seen in overlapping chains of experience memories, in continued beliefs, desires, intentions, and particularly in the carrying out of intentions, as well as in enduring personality traits (pp.205, 207).

Parfit (1984) distinguishes personal identity from Relation R as follows. Strong connectedness (an essential aspect of Relation R) is not transitive. X is strongly connected to him/herself yesterday, but not to him/herself forty years ago; and X 10 years hence is not as strongly connected to X now, as X now is to X tomorrow. Personal identity, on the other hand, is transitive. X is X now and was X 40 years ago and will be X in 10 years.

identity, it is more important. This too is usually unproblematic for Person D as Relation R and personal identity almost always are concurrent.

However, then there are the cases when they do not coincide. Here is one situation, the 'Branch-Line case' as Parfit (1984, pp.200–201) imagines it: Teletransportation has been *improved* such that Earth-D will no longer be destroyed. Person D is informed of this on his latest trip, but only after he has already pressed the button thereby initiating his teletransportation. D immediately realizes that his earthly and mars-ly counterparts will soon coexist and even communicate, suddenly raising a big problem. He, now (on Earth) feels his personal identity is as Earth-D; however, Mars-D will also identify himself as D. Moreover, Mars-D will be fully psychologically connected, and absolutely continuous with Earth-D, to all appearance identical. But can there be two of him? Now as if that did not complicate things enough, D is next told that the new technology has failed in a peculiar way; D is made aware that although indeed his body (a.k.a. Earth-D) will not be rendered unconscious and immediately destroyed in the usual fashion, he will suffer a slow cardiac death in a few days. Will this change how Earth-D feels about Mars-D as a continuation of himself? In any case, in a few days there will no longer be two Ds, but the one remaining will be Mars-D.

With the old teletransport system, D's life could plausibly be construed as progressing along one main line; Person D went from Earth-D to Mars-D. However, with the advent of the so-called improved technology, D's life could continue along two branches simultaneously. Both Earth-D and Mars-D would exist; and they would overlap. True with the spectacular technical failure of the new procedure, only Mars-D will continue to exist, as Earth-D will die; but this will follow a possible troubling, albeit short, period of overlap.

These imagined events raise several philosophical problems: First, for those who initially regarded Mars-D as a continuation of Person D, can they still regard him as such when there is an overlap with Earth-D? If they can, they are left with the problem of D being more than one person. In addition, how can something that is numerically identical—Person D is identical to himself—be two entities? If this problem abates for them when Earth-D dies—for then Mars-D will be the sole Person D—they must account for a serious

---

'Because identity is a transitive relation, the criterion of identity must also be a transitive relation. Since strong connectedness [Relation R] is not transitive, it cannot be the criterion of identity' (p.206). In other words, Relation R is not only different from personal identity, it cannot be the criterion by which identity is determined. (As is described later in the section, Parfit asserts further that it is Relation R, more than personal identity, with which he is concerned when he is concerned with his own survival.)

inconsistency: how can contingent matters affecting Earth-D alone entirely change the status of Mars D-as identical with Person D?

Clearly, these Branch-Line issues are much like those discussed above in the subsections on fission, both for amoebas and humans. They are well recognized by the various philosophers discussed in this chapter—Parfit (1984, pp.261–266), Wiggins (1979), Williams (1960/1973), and Nozick (1981, Part I, Chapter 1) —with Nozick (1981, p.32) summing up the situation thus: '… identity cannot depend upon whether there is or isn't another thing of a certain sort; …if there could be another thing so then there would not be identity, then there isn't identity, even if that other thing does not actually exist.'

However, according to Parfit (1984, pp. 202–209; 231–243), things are no simpler for those who did not ever regard Mars-D as a continuation of Earth-D. Noting that a butterfly developing into a caterpillar is a naturally occurring example of a numerically identical creature, yet one that is very different in each stage, Parfit considers questions about the limits of what can constitute a person's continuance as the same person. Suppose that cells from Earth-D were replaced with the material from which Mars-D's brain was to be constructed not only one neuron at a time, but very slowly. Would the gradual-versus-the-sudden replacement change those who viewed Earth-D and Mars-D as only 'exactly similar' to a position on which they were now 'numerically identical'? Or a simpler question, how many replacement parts can something endure and still be the original?[17]

Personhood, Parfit concludes, seems to be determined by 1) physical criteria, amounting to spatio-temporal physical continuity of at least the brain and at most the brain and body, and/or 2) psychological criteria, with this later comprising Relation R—psychological continuity and psychological connectedness.[18] However, then Parfit takes a very interesting turn. Using the notion of spectra—physical, psychological, and combined—Parfit demonstrates with sorites arguments (see this volume, Chapter 3) that all of the concepts involved in evaluating personhood are hopelessly vague. Would you accept that someone *is* still you, if 10% of your brain had been removed, and you were left with 90% of your original physical make-up, and 90% of your psychology? You can also ask the question this way: Is a person who is 90% you, both physically and

---

[17] These questions make it clear that 'self,' 'identity,' and even 'entity' are vague. More on this follows just below and see Chapter 3, this volume, for extensive discussions on vagueness.

[18] For Parfit, Relation R, although psychological in nature, is itself physically based, specifically brain based. On Parfit's account whatever is important in one's psychology—one's intentions, desires, goals, personality, etc.—all of this is caused by brain goings-on.

psychologically, *you*? What about 88% or 85%? And then there is this further question: Does the person who is 85% of your physical being and 85% of your psychology still the 'you' you want to survive when you care about your survival? What about 80% or 75%? If you accept 75%, what about 68%? And so forth. What Parfit shows is that there is no clear, coherent concept of person, using physical, psychological, or combined measures.

We are left with two linked problems: 1) the fission problem—when what I care about is my own survival, how can there be two of 'me'? And 2) the vagueness problem—how can I demarcate what constitutes 'me,' when the concept is vague, physically and psychologically? Parfit (1984) has an original solution that works for both problems. He suggests (pp.233, 235, 241–243), that although we want to think of our identity as determinate, and we want to be able to answer questions like: 'Am I going to die in the teletransporter?' and 'Is that person me or not me?'—these questions are empty and wrong. To remedy this, he suggests that when I am interested in my survival, I should be less concerned with perpetuating my particular singular personal identity and more concerned about the survival of all and anybody (anything) with Relation R to me. If my psychological continuity and connectedness continues, it does not matter if I have undergone fission and there are two (or even more) of me. Relatedly, I do not have to specify with precision what (who) would count as someone with my personal identity, i.e., the 'same person as I am.' Instead, given that I am concerned with my own survival, I should be increasingly concerned with the survival of those who have more Relation R to me; and I should still have some interest in anyone who has some (or any) Relation R to me, etc. In other words, for Parfit, the matter is relatively straightforward and not that complicated: My concern with my own survival should essentially be a concern with the survival of all Xs that bear Relation R to me; and my concern with any particular X should vary positively as a function of that X's increased Relation R to me.

Note that in Parfit's solution to the dilemmas of the survival of 'me'-ness, *personal identity* is supplanted by *Relation R*. This is interesting, and so is its consequence—that singularity no longer has importance. Nozick, whose views we will take up next, also treats the singularity aspect of 'me'-ness in an unusual fashion.

Closest continuer

For Nozick (1981, pp. 33–70) it is our *closest continuer* about which we are concerned, when we are interested in our own survival. However, if we have no closest continuer, but instead have *close enough continuers*, we can care about these just about as much.

Defining the closest continuer, Nozick (1981, p.34) explains: 'The closest continuer view presents a necessary condition for identity; something at t_2 is not the same entity as x at t_1 if it is not x's closest continuer. And "closest" means closer than all the others. If two things tie [in their closeness to x]...then neither is the same entity as x.' Nozick next points out that while closest continuer status is necessary for identity constitution, it is not sufficient: '... something may be the closest continuer of x without it being close enough to be x' (p.34).

Nozick goes on to describe several interesting thought experiment cases, variations on those with which we are familiar involving transplanted brains and hemi-brains, cloned bodies, dying original bodies, and replicas with psychological continuity. What is interesting in Nozick's examples is that, depending on the circumstance, the very same person-entity that is considered the closest continuer in one situation will certainly not be the closest continuer in another. To illustrate, take Parfit's teletransportation type cases. As long as Earth-D is alive, Nozick asserts that Earth-D and not Mars-D, will be Person D's closest continuer. However, as soon as Earth-D is gone, either through immediate destruction in the original process of teletransportation, or via the slow, cardiac death days later caused by the new procedure, Mars-D becomes Person D's sole closest continuer. Nozick has in this way, with the context sensitivity of the closest continuer model, been able to solve elegantly several of the vexing dilemmas about 'my' survival that we have been considering. Earth-D is the *de facto* Person D until Earth-D is no more. Then Mars-D becomes Person D, despite the fact that this was not Mar-D's status just moments prior to Earth-D's destruction or death. When teletransporting Person D back to Earth, Mars-D ceases to be Person D as soon as Earth-D is back on the scene. If something goes awry and Earth-D is never reconstituted as such, Mars-D remains as Person D. Indeed, Nozick's solution works very well, particularly in addressing questions like the one articulated above—how can contingent matters affecting Earth-D alone entirely change the identity status of Mars-D with respect to Person D? Dilemmas such as these dissolve with Nozick's context-dependent closest continuer. However, the closest continuer model does face a serious problem when it comes to those cases in which there are ties as to which of two (or more) possibilities is someone's closest continuer.

'Y at t_2 and Z at t_2 continue X at t_1 equally closely, closely enough so that either, in the absence of the other, would be (part of the same continuing entity as) X at t_1' (Nozick 1981, p.62). Considering himself X and, no longer existing, given that there is no single closest continuer, Nozick (p.63) writes, 'I am neither Y nor Z, and I no longer exist. This is not distressing in this case, for what I care about is that there remains something that continues me closely enough to be me if it were my sole continuer; and if there are two such, I care especially about the fate of the [tied] closest continuer.' However, this suggests that the closest continuer *can* be two. But Nozick holds that neither identity over time nor personal identity can be two (p.68), and he has further stated (p.68): that 'the closest continuer better realizes identity than does the relation: tie with close enough continuers.' To further complicate matters, Nozick remarks several times (pp.64, 65, 67, 68) that although we care most about the closest continuer when one exists, we do not care all that much that there is one, as long as there are continuers that are close enough:

> [G]iven that we care about our identity, we care especially about our closest continuer when it exists, yet do not care especially that we have a closest continuer, provided we have close enough continuers. How is the tie case to be described on this view? I do not view a tie as like death; I am no longer there, yet it is a good enough realization of identity to capture my care which attaches to identity (Nozick, 1981, p.68).

What are we to conclude? Either Nozick is claiming that identity is not numerically singular despite the threat of incoherence and his own comments to the contrary, or he is claiming there is something else. This 'something else' might be an identity-like relation that 'is a good enough realization of identity' that does not require singularity. This would be present in closest continuer and no less in close-enough continuers to sufficiently constitute my 'me'-ness when I am concerned with my own future [19] survival.

There is something unsatisfying with this conclusion. For one thing it leaves open the possibility of 'type' and 'token' people. Described by Williams (1970/1973, pp.79–81) a particular type–person could have any number of tokens, all of whom could count as close-enough continuers. Here is how this would look. Take the brain of someone, LAWB. Now take all of its structure and information and transfer it cell-by-cell to a new brain; and put this new brain in a new body, built up also on the blueprint of LAWB. However, if this can be done once, it can be done *n*-number of times. This seems like a *reductio* argument against Nozick's position, as Nozick would have to claim that as the original LAWB, I, should be fine with this whole bevy of 'me'-tokens, and not especially prefer that I should continue as just one.

---

[19] Thomas Nagel (1986) points out that quite contrary to our almost universal desire for self survival in the future, we are not at all disturbed about our absence in the past world, before we were born. Calling it '…the most perplexing feature of our attitude toward death,' he points to 'the asymmetry between our attitudes toward past and future non-existence. We do not regard the period before we were born in the same way that we regard the prospect of death' (p.228).

Even if this were unproblematic, one would still have to wonder in cases like this with multiple and tied closest continuers, what exactly Nozick has in mind as being distinct from personal identity and identity over time and yet capable of instantiating identity well enough to (in his words, p.68) 'capture my care.' What is this identity-like concept?

Rather than trying to solve Nozick's problem in reconciling identity/'me'-ness with his version of non-singularity, let me suggest that the fact of his serious troubles on this score can prove highly instructive. In fact, in the next section, I take up 'me'-ness as necessarily singular, the efforts of Parfit and Nozick to the contrary notwithstanding. In order to make this case, I return to the psychoanalytic and other clinical and nonclinical examples as well as continuing with various philosophical dilemmas and accounts.

Agency: 'Me'-ness in the philosophical cases

The main claims I put forward in this section are: 1) it is our agency with which we are concerned when we are concerned about our own survival, just as it is agency that is at stake in the psychoanalytic and other cases; 2) in other words, agency *is* my 'me'-ness; 3) agency is necessarily singular; and 4) agency consists in intentional actions, with intentions defined broadly.

My agency, my 'me'-ness

When I want my own survival, what is the nature of this 'me' with which I am concerned? I propose the following answer: The 'me' whose survival interests me when I am concerned about my own survival is the 'me' who represents my agency. This answer leads of course to the next question—just what is agency, what is an agent? Most notable in any understanding of the characteristics and capacities of agents are their intentions and intentional acts; these predicated on their desires, beliefs, other psychological attitudes, and personality and character traits. Among the many desires I have, some are universal (or nearly so) as they are related to the drives striving to satisfy biological needs. When I am thirsty, I desire to drink; when hungry, I desire to eat, etc. In addition, along with (all?) other animals, I have the drive-derived desire to survive, this desire being the very one that fuels my concern about my own survival.[20] Note that these drive-derived desires, in particular, demonstrate clearly that my agency is different from my personhood. The latter is more sophisticated,

---

[20] Do I care that this particular desire, the desire to survive, survives? Probably, I do, as it is hard to imagine a biological agential creature lacking that desire (although this desire need not be conscious).

quite distinct from other animals' 'animal-hood,' and is perhaps best characterized by Frankfurt (1971/1988) as consisting in 'second-order volitions,' in
which a person wants his/her actions to be determined by one set of 'first-
order' desires rather than another.[21] My agency, on the other hand, predicated
on drive-derived desires common throughout the animal world, is closely tied
to action. The role of action in agency, along with a continued discussion
about agency's singularity, are the two central topics of this section. I take up
agency's singularity first.

Agency is singular

If I am correct that it is ourselves as agents about whom we are concerned when
we are interested in our own survival, and if I am correct that agency is singular,
we should see a problem with thinking of ourselves as more than one. Thomas
Nagel, even while questioning the correctness of his strong view that agents are
necessarily singular, highlights the problems with an alternative position.
Describing commisurectomy patients—those who have had their corpus
callosum severed, removing the bridge between one hemisphere of their brain
and the other, (owing to tumor or seizure)—Nagel admits that many seem to
function in a variety of circumstances as though with two separate conscious-
nesses. Despite this, Nagel *cannot* find agency anything other than singular,
even in these special cases, and therefore remarks, confused and confusingly:
'[W]e take ourselves as paradigms of psychological unity, and are then unable
to project ourselves into their lives, either once or twice' (Nagel, 1971/1975,
p.242). Later, Nagel (1986) better explicates his view as he comments on some
of the thought experiment cases discussed in the last section: 'If I am told that
my brain is about to be split, and that the left half will be miserable and the right
half euphoric, there is no form that my subjective expectations can take, because
my idea of myself doesn't allow for divisibility—nor do the emotions of expectation, fear and hope' (pp. 44–45). For Nagel his agency, the 'me'-ness whence
his subjective expectations, fears, and hopes arise, is necessarily singular.

David Wiggins (1979) stresses the animal instinct and, important for my
view, links it to singularity. 'The instinct for survival has played its part…But
what is the content of said instinct? The content is surely that this animal that
is [numerically] identical with *me* [his emphasis] should not cease to be but
should survive and flourish' (p.420). Discussing further the usual sorts of sub-
limated traces one can leave, living on in one's works, or having done some
lasting good, Wiggins (1979, p.422) could not be clearer about the singularity

---

[21] See Frankfurt (1971/1988, especially p.16). Also, see the subsection on 'Akrasia' earlier in
this chapter.

of that whom he cares about in terms of survival: 'What I am certain about is that I do not see how the offer of any of these things, Parfitian [Relation R descendants] or etiolated, can be taken for a proper surrogate (equivalent on the level of imagination, conception, and desire) for the continued existence of the one and only person that is me.'

Especially in conjunction with the problems of non-singularity in Nozick's work, the assertions of Wiggins and Nagel help my own view on the singularity front—that the 'me' of my survival means the survival over time of that one animal that is numerically identical with me. Still, I have much work to do to establish that it is my *agency* that I project into that singular being that I regard as the continuation of 'me.' So before even taking up the action aspect of agency promised above, let me offer a deeper investigation into the nature of agency.

But again, what is agency?

G.E.M. Anscombe (1957, p.9) asks the question: 'What distinguishes actions which are intentional from those which are not?' She responds to her own question: '...they are the actions to which a certain sense of the question "Why?" is given application; the sense is...the answer [to the question "Why?"]...gives a reason for [the] action.' Anscombe moreover considers this a necessary feature of intentional actions, '...the concept of ...intentional action would not exist, if the question "Why?", with answers that give reasons for acting, did not' (p.34).

These definitions of agency seem fine for language competent humans. However, I have held that the drive-desires that we share with animals are quite essential in our agency; indeed, in my view, animals are agents too. Anscombe (pp.86–87) also addresses this matter, concluding that the descriptions of many animal actions fit too well with descriptions of intentions not to be intentions. However, because of the work in evolutionary biology in the intervening decades, we can now also avail ourselves of a more complete understanding thanks to some basic concepts from that field.

To the extent that animals can have motives, intentions, and intentional actions of the sort we humans have, the question 'Why?' can be asked just as it can in the human case. But what about actions that are instinctually driven, but *appear* to be irrational, where it is evident that the standard 'Why?' question can have no useful application? Say, e.g., frogs' indiscriminately swallowing bugs *and* black metal BBs. A case like this reveals that for animals (and for us) motives, intentions, and actions have both *proximate* and *ultimate* explanations (Alcock, 2001, pp. 16, 130). The *proximate* explanations are those that answer the 'Why?' question in terms of volition. Why did the chicken cross the road? It wanted to get to the other side. In the *ultimate* explanations, answers to the 'Why?' questions are determined by evolutionary fitness rather than volition. So, why do frogs swallow all those metal BBs? Frog fitness has been enhanced by a swallowing mechanism that is triggered whenever an object of a certain description—one clearly fitting both bugs and BBs—is but a tongue's length away.[22]

With the question 'Why?' extended such that it can include evolutionarily causal explanations as well as volitional reasons, agency can be extended throughout the animal world, whenever there are actions to which one or the other application of 'Why?' can pertain. Thus, on my account, even amoebas (figuring so prominently in these discussions) should be viewed as agents, e.g., as they move to engulf or extrude. Why does amoeba X extrude that y-type particle now? On the evolutionary application of why, extruding particles of y-type has increased the fitness of amoebas. In addition, why does amoeba X divide now into daughters A and B? Again the evolutionary/ultimate explanation provides an answer in terms of the fitness success of X's genetic material if division occurs at a particular time when certain conditions obtain. In my view then, not only is it the case that amoebas are singular agents, but they are single agents whose last agential acts under normal conditions are those involving their own division.

We have talked of agency as singular, and agential actions as intentional in that they are actions to which the question 'Why?' in at least one of its forms can be applied and answered. Thus, now it is time to return to explore the action/movement aspect of agency.

Action in agency

Agency implies motivated motion, i.e., intentional action. Linking singularity, action, agency, and what amounts to the concern about my continued 'me'-ness, Stuart Hampshire (1959, pp.59–60, 67–69) first describes the initial conditions for being a person as entailing being a distinct physical entity who acts agentially on other objects and persons in the world.[23] Mirroring Anscombe

---

[22] Note that actions can admit of both proximate and ultimate explanations. For example, the chicken, crossing the road because it wants to, might want to especially because there is food or a potential mate, or because it is being chased by a predator, etc.

[23] For Hampshire, knowing oneself as a person, distinct from other persons and objects, first entails noting the effects of one's own agential actions. (This seems a very Kantian idea [from the *Critique of Pure Reason* (1781/1787)], where the unity of the self rests upon the self as the perceiver of the unity of objects, while the unity of an object is known only through the several percepts of it all possessed by the same perceiving self.)

Note that Bernard Williams (1956–57/1973, p.4) similarly uses action as a criterion for individuating agents (although he too uses the word 'persons'): 'Any token event E, and any

Hampshire (1959) claims, '"With a view to", or "in order to", are unavoidable idioms in giving the sense of the notion of an action, the arrow of agency passing through the present and pointing forward in time' (p.73). Moreover, for Hampshire (1959), the body is not just an instrument of intentional acts (pp.79–80); rather the body is the intention-in-action, such that when an action is animated by an agent's intentions, 'there is no reason to look for some criterion of personal identity that is distinct from our bodies as persisting physical objects' (p.74–75). In other words, our personal identity is no more and no less than our agential intentions, these intentions necessarily instantiated in our physical bodies. Finally, putting agency at the center of Relation R type psychological continuity too, Hampshire (1959, p.72) states, '...we carry our intentions with us, and this carrying forward of intentions, together with the perception of movement, provides the natural and necessary continuity of our experience.'

Writing at about the same time as Hampshire (but with very different philosophical goals),[24] P.F. Strawson comes to similar conclusions regarding action and agency. Strawson's (1959) work is a quest for a descriptive metaphysics of 'individuals,' both material entities and persons. Dividing up the world into the predicates pertaining to persons, P-predicates, and those pertaining to the material realm, M-predicates, Strawson (1959, p.104) discusses the problem of how P-predicates are even possible: '...a beginning can be made by moving a certain class of P-predicates to a central position...They are predicates...which involve doing something, which clearly imply intention...and which indicate a characteristic pattern...of bodily movement' (p.111). I take Strawson to be talking of agency here, despite his use of the term 'person' as he is at this point not requiring anything of his P-predicates beyond simple intentional activity.

From a totally different philosophical quarter, Maurice Merleau-Ponty (1962, p.137) in his *Phenomenology of Perception* presents a similar take on agency, desire, and action, in a section in which he considers the role of our own movements in the development of concepts of space: 'Consciousness is in the first place not a matter of "I think" but of "I can".' This phrase is commented upon by A.J. Ayer (1982) who agrees with Merleau-Ponty and adds, '...this implies...that we enter the world as [active] agents as well as observers, and that what we attend to may at the most primitive level be a function of what we desire...' (pp.218–219).

---

token action A, are by definition particulars. Moreover, the description "the man who did the action A" necessarily individuates some one person; for it is logically impossible that two persons should do the same *token* [his emphasis] action.'

[24] Hampshire's (1959) book concerns moral philosophy, in particular free will.

More on action and agency: Biological foundations

In this chapter I have been making the case for action as a necessary component of agency, stressing that animals, including amoebas, acting intentionally (given that intentional is understood also in its evolutionary ultimate sense), are agents too. Here (and in prior work) I have also held that desires, particularly those that are close to the drives from which all desires are derived, are central to actions. Specifically, I have argued that desire has the constitutive function of the 'willingness (and readiness) to act toward its own fulfillment.' (See Brakel, 2009, Chapter 8.)

Howard Shevrin (2003), who has developed a view of agency not far from my own, [25] similarly locates a particular part of a drive, its 'pressure' or 'motor factor'—that which Freud (1915, p.122) characterized as '...the amount of force or the measure of the demand for work which it [the drive] represents'—as the central factor both in action and agency. Shevrin (2003, p.13), '...propose[s] that this pressure...is at the heart of what we mean by agency, the foundation for the...self as *actor* [his emphasis].' Then Shevrin (p.13) does something quite important, proposing that 'From a neurophysiological and neuroanatomical standpoint agency appears to be instantiated in a particular brain circuitry characterized by a particular neurotransmitter.' Shevrin refers to the 'SEEKING system' of Jaak Panksepp (Panksepp 1998, chapter 8, pp.144–163), consisting of dopaminergic (DA)[26] circuits in the lateral hypothalamic corridor from the ventral tegmental area (VTA) to the nucleus accumbens septi (NAS) of the brain (Panksepp, 1998, p.145). Panksepp (p.145) describes the reaction in animals upon electrical stimulation of this area as '...the most energized exploratory and search behaviors an animal is capable of exhibiting.' As this SEEKING system activity is not linked to a specific drive, and because (chemically) blocking the DA NAS/SEEKING system circuitry causes inertia even under conditions of need, Shevrin (2003, p.13) suggests that its activation is 'a pure culture of agency,' that the 'urge to move, to act is the most primitive and abiding aspect of animal life.' He goes on to say 'Self-initiated movement and action *is* agency [his emphasis].'

---

[25] This is not surprising. We have worked very closely for more than 25 years; much of the time with Shevrin as the director and myself as co-associate director of the Hunt Memorial Laboratory for the Study of Unconscious Processes at the University of Michigan. Ideas in the laboratory were fluid; and although I believe my views on agency are my own, deriving from my philosophical studies as well as research investigations, no doubt they were influenced by Shevrin's, as his were by mine.

[26] Dopamine is a neurotransmitter.

I take issue with him here, for on my view agents must not only act, but act in such a way that one or another version of the question 'Why' must be applicable.[27] We are, however, certainly in agreement that all animals are capable of agent-driven actions. More significantly, Shevrin's insight has provided reason to believe that the motor aspect of agential action has a specific brain-based biological foundation.

Panksepp's SEEKING system, both in neuroanatomy and neurophysiology, maps quite well onto the 'wanting' system of Kent Berridge. Berridge and his colleague Terry Robinson (Robinson and Berridge,1993; Berridge and Robinson,1998,2003, 2008) have shown that this 'wanting' system is quite separable from the so-called 'liking' system, although both systems play a role in the experience of reward. Berridge (1996, p.1) states that the two systems '... can be manipulated and measured separately;' that 'Liking and wanting have separable neural substrates;' and that 'Both liking and wanting can exist without subjective awareness.'

This last point, asserting that there can be unconscious liking and unconscious desiring (i.e., unconscious wanting), is of particular interest because it supports the psychoanalytic claim that desires, and with them various aspects of an agential agenda, can indeed be unconscious. This is of importance in the next section where we take up two new potential problems regarding the singularity of agency—the first problem occasioned by psychoanalytic cases.

Is agency really singular?

I have made much of the view that agency is the 'me'-ness I care about when I am concerned about my survival, and that the agency in question, predicated on desire and action, is necessarily singular. On this view, agency is not projectable into multiple embodied selves, no matter how R-Related they are. Agency only exists singularly as the continuation of that me-over-time, numerically identical with me (i.e., the original me).

However, two types of cases raise potential problems with my account of agency as singular. First, from the psychoanalytic domain there are clinical and nonclinical cases in which people seem to have such very conflicted agential agendas along with multi-directional behaviors, that one is at least advised to question the singular view of agency. Second, there are the biological cases, the so-called superorganisms, observed in anthills, bee hives, and termite mounds, in which the whole colony, rather than each individual creature, appears to be the singular agent.

---

[27] In other words, my account of agency is more constrained: it allows that not every action, but only those actions to which the question 'Why?' in either of its version can apply. (See this chapter pp.121–122.)

I take up the psychoanalytic type cases first. Here, I maintain that appearances to the contrary notwithstanding, agency *is* singular.

Psychoanalytic (and other, nonclinical) cases

Dr. M and others

Dr. M was a woman in her late 20s who was a very ambitious linguist. Her work was going well, but with foreign expeditions, and academic writings, she had almost no time for a personal life. She had ambivalent feelings about this; she wanted someday to be married and possibly to have children, but certainly not anytime soon. Although she did not have a steady partner, she had a diaphragm, as she was occasionally sexually active. Then Dr. M met a man she really liked, F. F was a successful scholar in English literature, a man in his mid-30s, who was eager to settle down in the very near future. This meant he wanted to marry and have kids as soon as possible. Dr. M really liked F, but still felt a long way from wanting any part of settling down. Despite this, probably owing to a single lapse in her use of the diaphragm (which with effort she could almost remember), some 4 months into their relationship, 5 weeks after she and F had started living together, Dr. M was startled to find that the 'weird' symptoms she had been experiencing were diagnosed as those to be expected in a normal first pregnancy. She did not know what to do. She liked F, and thought he would be a fine husband and father, but she did not want to marry now, much less have a child. And yet, would a man better fit for being her mate come her way?

As she wrestled with herself as to whether or not to have an abortion, Dr. M had an experience made much more comprehensible owing to the Berridge and Robinson findings establishing a distinction between wanting and liking systems. Dr. M felt strong cravings for foods she did not even like, this occurring almost every day in the first several weeks after she learned she was pregnant. Moreover, she felt impelled to act on these desires, procuring whatever food she wanted but did not like. This so far is not unlike what many pregnant women experience. For Dr. M, however, the fracture between her cravings/wantings on the one hand, and her preferences/likings on the other, was very hard for her to tolerate. Before her pregnancy she liked what she desired, especially with respect to food, and so acting on those desires seemed natural. Now, being driven to act on desires for items she did not like made her feel 'alien to herself.' She said she felt that 'something, perhaps the fetus, is directing me and my actions in directions different from what *I* want.' This was not made any easier by her 'intuition' that F really wanted her to have the baby. Although she admitted that he never really said as much, she felt he was hiding his real feelings, instead being politically correct and careful.

Dr. M's reaction to this situation can best be described using psychoanalytic concepts, particularly unconscious desire and unconscious agency, concepts that will also help demonstrate that Dr. M's agency is singular, even when it may seem plural. Dr. M felt ambivalent about every aspect of her pregnancy. On the side of wanting *not to be pregnant*: She wanted to continue her career unburdened, and she wished she had used her diaphragm. Most of the time Dr. M acted on these conscious desires. Yet there were other desires, conscious and unconscious on the side of wanting to *be pregnant*. She wanted to continue her relationship with F. Further, she felt that F strongly desired her to want to marry and have children soon, and she wanted to please him. She herself wanted children, someday. Most tellingly, she forgot to insert her diaphragm, indicating that on that day at that time it was plausible to infer that she had an unconscious desire to become pregnant, *right then*. The unconscious desire to become pregnant, like all desires, has as its constitutive function a readiness to act toward its fulfillment, and in this case the act of forgetting was the action occasioned by the unconscious desire.

So what we have so far is Dr. M with conflicted desires, some conscious and some unconscious. Indeed, single agents often have such conflicted desires. Since every intentional act is by definition agent driven, and since a great many acts are the result of rapid and automatic unconscious mental calculation, weighing the various conflicting desires, and considering other factors such as the likelihood and consequence of fulfillment, one can reasonably conclude that many of the agential acts of single agents result from syntheses of conflicting desires. So was the case for Dr. M, with respect to getting pregnant and so will be the case for Dr. M with respect to her ultimate decisions about the pregnancy.[28]

From a long-range point of view too, single agents have many agential agendas. Sometimes, compromise syntheses take place as above; sometimes, there are alterations between agendas. During my own 10th year, I wanted both to be a grown-up male baseball player and a little girl. Recognizing these two conflicting agential agendas, my parents gave me two birthday presents—a real major league hardball glove and a very cute stuffed animal, a yellow puppy-dog. That same year for Halloween I had two costumes, representing two further agential developments. For half of that day I wore a costume in which I looked like a very serious woman doctor, and for the other half I dressed as a flashy feminine Spanish dancer. Instead of the single event syntheses described

---

[28] Note also that symptoms and dreams arise on a similar basis, with the resultant manifest dream or psychological symptom representing not only different, but often conflicting wishes and desires, along with defenses against at least some of them, all in a condensed and displaced form, expressing and disguising these unconscious wishes and desires.

above, in these longer term conflicts, one agential agenda gets enacted and then the other. One of the key tasks of adolescence, not unlike that of a good analysis, is to work out a more consistent sense of agency with less radical conflicts, but one allowing diverse agential aims. In any case, both the short-term compromise syntheses and the longer range alternation of agential agendas, take place within a single agent.

Returning then to Dr. M, it is not that her two sets of conflicted desires regarding her pregnancy *did* represent two different agents, but rather she experienced herself as two agents, with 'something' inside of her driving the actions that she felt to be at war with her own volition.[29] Further, Dr. M, unconscious of *her own agential* desires to be and stay pregnant, not only rendered this aspect of her singular agency unconscious, she projected it onto F.

The psychoanalytic and other clinical and nonclinical cases, despite initial impressions, do not present any threat to the view that agency is singular. The challenge to this view of agency is more daunting from the biological world of superorganisms.

Agency in superorgansims

Many have argued (or assumed) that the boundaries of an agent are those boundaries defining the discrete body of an animal.[30] Whether that boundary consists in the cell membrane of a single-celled creature or the more complex outer coverings of multicellular animals, it functions as a barrier to keep the inside of an animal intact, differentiating the animal from the world outside of it. Although I continue to find this definition of singular agents appealing as applied throughout the animal world, I must admit that the superorganisms do provide a compelling counterexample.

---

[29] Dr. M's agential drive to procure and eat the various foods she craved but did not like represent on a psychological and biological level her unconscious desire to keep the pregnancy. However, note these strange cravings also represent a strictly biological and totally unconscious desire for survival. It is as though her body were saying, 'These foods have elements necessary for survival, given this extra physiological load.'

On a much more speculative level, given my own view in which agency includes even single-celled beings, the possibility that some sort of biological competition for resources between the fetus and Dr. M as the pregnant provider cannot be ruled out. If this indeed is the case, Dr. M's experience of two agencies might in some part reflect the contribution of this strictly biological reality.

[30] For example, to name just those discussed within this chapter, David Wiggins, Bernard Williams, Thomas Nagel, Howard Shevrin, and I (L.A.W. Brakel) all hold this view.

To introduce the concept of superorganism, I quote at some length Edward O. Wilson, ant expert, and eminent biologist:

> The vast majority of insect, verterbrate, and other animal populations evolve primarily through selection at the level of individual organism…In the advanced social insects,[31] in contrast, selection occurs primarily at the level of the colony, with workers mostly or entirely eliminated from reproduction and colonies competing against one another as compact units…the workers will increase the replication of genes identical to their own by promoting the physical well-being of the colony, even if they sacrifice themselves to achieve this end (1985, p.1490).

E.O. Wilson (p.1492) continues, 'The workers of advanced insect societies are not unlike cells that emigrate to new positions, transform into new types, and aggregate to form tissues and organs.'

Although the concept of superorganism is not without its detractors, David Sloane Wilson and Eliot Sober (1989, p.337) find that the evidence against the concept rests on a combination of theoretical confusion and rigidity (pp.337–338). Agreeing with E.O. Wilson, they claim that a 'Collection of individuals can become functionally organized by natural selection, in exactly that way that individuals themselves become functionally organized' (p.338). Defining 'organism' as a life form in which mutually dependent parts maintain its vital functions, D.S. Wilson and Sober (1989, p.339) then define 'superorganism.' A superorganism is '… a collection of single creatures that together possess the functional organization implicit in the formal definition of organism' (p.339). They continue (p.339): 'Just as genes and organs do not qualify as organisms, the single creatures that make up a superorganism also may not qualify as organisms in the formal sense of the word.'

Continuing with findings that necessitate some adjustment to any universal notion of agency bounded by an individual creature's boundaries, Seely (1989) discusses the world of honeybees. 'A colony of honey bees, for example, functions as an integrated whole and its members cannot survive on their own, yet individual honey bees are physically independent and closely resemble in physiology and morphology the solitary bees from which they evolved' (pp.546–548). Seely explains (pp.449–551) that these bees are not given instructions from the queen. Instead, they are sensitive to biological cues that indicate, e.g., bio-mass of fellow bees of different developmental stages at specific hive areas, and honey storage capacity at specific times, both of these 'dictating' a variety of different worker bee assignments and actions, all as a function of the quantitative amounts registered. The lack of 'centralized

---

[31] Advanced social insects that are thought to be superorganisms include leaf-cutter ants, fungus-growing termites, and honey bees [my footnote].

decision making' even by the queen (p.549), and the 'coordinated group action' at the level of the colony (p.551), certainly suggest that the whole hive is the agent that drives honeybee actions, rather than any individual bee.

While I might be able to launch some argument for my view to the effect that the group-actions of individuals in a superorganism remain actions such that the 'Why?' question can be answered by the evolutionary explanation of selection forces—in this way not unlike the acts of single cellular creatures—I am not inclined to and do not intend to do this. Why? Because the individual bees, ants, and termites, like particular cells in a multicellular organism, submit to routine sacrifice. Each bee, ant, and termite, like each cell in a multicellular creature *does* play a part in helping the genes of the colony (i.e., the multicellular individual) perpetuate themselves, but *does not* appear to answer the evolutionary question 'Why?' in terms of its own survival.[32] Further, the desire to survive is an essential constituent of an agent's agency; a necessary part of the 'me'-ness I am concerned with when I am concerned with my survival.

Summary

In this chapter I have put forth the view that agency is central to understanding 'me'-ness in a variety of situations. In the psychoanalytic realm (including clinical, and nonclinical settings) ubiquitous problems characterized as involving 'the self,' 'the ego,' or various defenses against drives, can be more deeply understood if they are conceptualized as problems of agency. I also discussed agency and the sense of 'me'-ness in the virtual world of 'Second Life' and agency in dreams, these as a prelude to exploring the philosophical dilemma of what constitutes the 'me' that I am concerned about, when I am concerned with my own survival. The views of several philosophers were presented and contrasted, resulting in the surprising conclusion that the 'me' whose survival I care about, is the 'me' of agency; the same agential 'me' involved in the many conflicts abounding in the psychoanalytic domain.

I derived and described my own account of agency, which includes the following: Agency is 1) singular (*pace* Parfit and Nozick), 2) it consists of our most important desires, which are in turn essentially linked to action, 3) agency implies intentional actions, with intentional defined as capable of answering 'Why?' questions in terms of a psychological and/or evolutionary explanation. Finally, 4) agency features in all animals, even single-celled individuals.

---

[32] As Seely describes just above, individual honeybees can be physically independent, and indeed, away from the colony individuals do act in order to survive, e.g., by avoiding predators. Nonetheless, within the colony the individuals are not each self-sufficient; and the actions of individuals serve colony survival at their own expense.

In line with this last, I presented some neuroanatomical and neurophysiological evidence for a biological foundation for agency as action.

Finally, challenging my own account, I raised two sorts of problems for the notion of agency as singular—psychoanalytic and biological. The psychoanalytic problem with multiple agential aims and agendas, I found on further exploration, to present no problem; the biological problem concerning agency in superorganisms remains intriguingly unsolved.

Conclusions

Perhaps more so than the other chapters in this book, this chapter on agency reveals the pure pleasure of discovery that can arise from doing interdisciplinary work. If one were to work solely as a psychoanalyst with psychoanalytic patients demonstrating that their deepest conflicts arise when they ask: 'What do *I* want to do with *my* life?' or solely as a philosopher grappling with the philosophical problem: 'What is the essence of the *me* I care about when I am concerned with my own survival?,' one's power to explore would likely be curtailed by each discipline's requirements and conventions. On the other hand, looking at the psychoanalytic cases and the philosophical question together, applying understanding gained from one field to the dilemmas of the other, new vistas become possible.

I am under no illusion that this chapter will change standard psychoanalytic practice by arguing that agency problems are central in most psychoanalytic patients' conflicts. Nor do I think that identifying the 'me' of concern when I am concerned with my own survival, as my agency, will turn the philosophy of action on its head. Rather, by discovering that in each domain a similar concept of agency can resolve certain vexing problems, an intellectual excitement can be generated, fueled by the convergent solution—a solution that in turn promises to advance and deepen the understanding of agency. Arising in just these circumstances, my own account of agency, because of its dual-disciplinary parentage, not only fully respects both disciplines, but also has the unique potential to expand both philosophical and psychoanalytic understanding of the agential 'me.'

References

Alcock, S (2001). *The Triumph of Sociobiology*. Oxford, Oxford University Press.

Anscombe, GEM (1957). *Intention*. Cambridge, Mass and London, Harvard University Press.

Ayer, AJ (1982). *Philosophy in the Twentieth Century*. New York, Vintage Books.

Berridge, K (1996). Food reward: brain substrates of wanting and liking. *Neuroscience and Biobehavioral Reviews*, **20**, 1–25.

Berridge, K and Robinson, T (1998). What is the role of dopamine in reward: hedonic impact, reward learning, or incentive salience? *Brain Research Reviews*, **28**, 309–369.

Berridge, K and Robinson, T (2003). Parsing reward. *Trends in Neuoroscience*, **26**, 507–513.

Berridge, K and Robinson, T (2008).The mind of an addicted brain: neural sensitization of wanting versus liking. *Current Directions in Psychological Science*, **4**, 71–75.

Brakel, LAW (2009). *Philosophy, Psychoanalysis, and the A-Rational Mind*. Oxford, Oxford University Press.

Brakel, LAW (2004). Ego constriction. *The American Journal of Psychoanalysis*, **64**, 267–277.

de Sousa, R (1976). Rational homunculi. In A Rorty, ed. *The Identity of Persons*, Chapter 9, 217–238. Berkeley and Los Angeles, University of California Press.

Frankfurt, H (1971/1988). Freedom of the will and the concept of a person. In *The Importance of What We Care About*, Chapter 2, 11–25. Cambridge, Cambridge University Press.

Frankfurt, H (1976). Identification and externality. In A Rorty, ed. *The Identity of Persons*, Chapter 10, 239–251. Berkeley and Los Angeles, University of California Press.

Freud, S (1900). *The Interpretation of Dreams*. Standard Edition, Vol. 4 & 5. Trans. and ed. J. Strachey. London, 1953, Hogarth Press.

Freud, S (1915). *Instincts and their Vicissitudes*. Standard Edition, Vol. 14. Trans. and ed. J. Strachey. London, 1957, Hogarth Press.

Hampshire, S (1959). *Thought and Action*. New York, Viking Press.

Kant, I (1781, 1787). *Critique of Pure Reason*. trans. Norman Kemp Smith. New York, 1965, St. Martin's Press.

Lewis, D (1976). Survival and identity. In A Rorty, ed. *The Identity of Persons*, Chapter 1, 17–40. Berkeley and Los Angeles, University of California.

Merleau-Ponty, M (1962). *Phenomenology of Perception*. Trans. Colin Smith. London, Routledge and Kegan Paul.

Nagel, T (1986). *The View from Nowhere*. Oxford and New York, Oxford University Press.

Nozick, R (1981). *Philosophical Explanations*. Cambridge, Mass, Harvard University Press.

Panksepp, J (1998). SEEKING systems and anticipatory states of the nervous system. In *Affective Neuroscience: The Foundation of Human and Animal Emotions*. Chapter 8, 144–163. New York, Oxford University Press.

Parfit, D (1984). *Reasons and Persons*. Oxford, Clarendon Press.

Penelhum, T (1955/1970). Hume on personal identity. In H.Morick, ed. *Introduction to the Philosphy of Mind*, 57–73. Glenview, Illinois, Scott, Foresman, and Co.

Penelhum, T (1971). The importance of self-identity. *The Journal of Philosophy*, **68**, 667–678.

Prior, AN (1965–1966). Existence and identity. *Proceedings of the Aristotelian Society*, **66**, 183–192.

Robinson, T and Berridge, K (1993). The neural basis of drug craving: an incentive-sensitization theory of addiction. *Brain Research Reviews*, **18**, 247–291.

Seely, T (1989). The honey bee colony as a superorganism. *American Scientist*, **77**, 546–553.

Shevrin, H (2003). The psychoanalytic theory of drive in the light of recent neuroscience findings and theories. Wilson Memorial Lecture, September 15, New York University, New York, New York.

Shoemaker, S (1963). *Self-Knowledge and Self-Identity*. Ithaca, New York, Cornell University Press.

Strawson, PF (1959). *Individuals*. London and New York, Routledge.

Velleman, JD (2008). Bodies, selves. *American Imago*, **65**, 405–426.

Wiggins, D (1967). *Identity and Spatio-temporal Continuity*. Oxford, Blackwell.

Wiggins, D (1979). The concern to survive. *Midwest Studies in Philosophy*, **4**, 417–422.

Williams, B (1956–1957/1973). Personal identity and individuation. In *Problems of the Self*, Chapter 1, 1–18. Cambridge, Cambridge University Press.

Williams, B (1960/1973). Bodily continuity and personal identity. In *Problems of the Self*, Chapter 2, 19–25. Cambridge, Cambridge University Press.

Williams, B (1970/1973). The self and the future. In *Problems of the Self*, Chapter 4, 46–63. Cambridge, Cambridge University Press.

Wilson, DS and Sober E (1989). Reviving the superorganism. *Journal of Theoretical Biology*, **136**, 337–356.

Wilson, EO (1985). The sociogenesis of insect colonies. *Science*, **228**, 1489–1495.

Part V

Placebo effect

Psychoanalytic theory

Chapter 5

The placebo effect: Psychoanalytic theory can help explain the phenomenon[1]

Prior to introducing this chapter, I want to point out to the reader that, unlike the previous chapters, this one will contain little new in the way of psychoanalytic theory and even less content from philosophy of mind and action. Instead, this chapter, focusing on an explanation for the placebo effect, is an instantiation of some principles quite relevant to the philosophy of science.[2] In fact, an evaluation of the explanation offered in this chapter will be taken up, both in particular and in the larger context of the nature of explanations in general, in the next and final chapter, 'Explanations and conclusions.'

Introduction

In the late 1970s and early 1980s Aldolf Grunbaum's (1977,1981,1982) view of psychoanalysis as a non-science was hotly contested. (See Marshall Edelson, 1984.) Although not claiming that psychoanalysis was ineffective, Grunbaum held its successes were attributable to suggestion and the placebo effect—nonspecific treatment measures—rather than the causal effect of psychoanalytic treatment. Grunbaum's basic challenge to psychoanalysis as a scientific discipline held that 1) psychoanalysis as a treatment was centrally predicated upon overcoming repression such that patient and analyst would agree on the contents uncovered—the so-called Tally argument; and 2) that the data so generated in the process of psychoanalysis could not be probative as these were a) contaminated by suggestion and b) not subject to scientific test as the data

---

[1] This article is a revised version of Brakel (2007). The placebo effect: Can psychoanalytic theory help explain the phenomenon? *American Imago*, Vol. 64, 273–281.

[2] An important critique of psychoanalysis as a science, as well as a response will be addressed in this chapter, albeit briefly, as these matters are tangential to the central argument advanced here, namely that aspects of psychoanalytic theory can play an explanatory role in understanding the placebo effect. (For a fuller defense of psychoanalysis as a science see Brakel, 2009, Chapters 1 and 2.)

were enumeratively inductive (i.e., here is another example bearing out X hypothesis) rather than eliminatively inductive (i.e., this result shows that X hypothesis cannot be correct, but Y hypothesis still stands).

There are two different sorts of answers to Grunbaum's challenges. As to his first claim, few psychoanalytic theorists hold that the central task in psychoanalysis is overcoming repression such that patient and analyst agree upon the reconstructed contents. To the extent that this is not central to psychoanalysis, the Tally argument against psychoanalysis rests on a faulty premise. With regard to the second claim, although in my view Grunbaum is correct that data presuming the assumptions (or hypotheses) under test cannot provide evidence for those assumptions, it is quite possible to conduct research on the assumptions of psychoanalysis with data outside the psychoanalytic situation, data that can be probative regarding these assumptions.[3] Furthermore, it is now widely recognized that theories based on eliminative induction are not the only sort of bona fide scientific theories. (This last point is discussed at length in Chapter 6, 'Explanations and conclusions.')

Despite this, twenty to thirty years after these debates, Grunbaum's critique continues to stimulate much that is of interest. For example, the question of the role of the placebo effect in psychoanalysis can hardly be said to be resolved. However, here there is the larger puzzle: the role of the placebo effect in psychoanalysis is unresolved, because the nature of the placebo effect—specifically, its psychological mechanisms—is itself unresolved. Thus, the purpose of this small chapter: I shall argue that irrespective of the role placebos play in successful psychoanalyses, psychoanalytic theory can help explain the psychological operations underlying placebo effects.

General findings and explanations

In the typical type of evaluation of new drugs or procedures, double-blind studies are conducted in which one group of randomly assigned subjects gets the active agent under test, another group gets an older reliable active agent, and a third group gets a placebo drug—with neither subjects nor experimenters knowing which individuals get which treatments. In the very best studies 1) the placebos are 'active,' which means that the placebo treatments have side

---

[3] See, e.g., the considerable body of work done at the Hunt Laboratory at the University of Michigan by Howard Shevrin, Linda A.W. Brakel, and Michael Snodgrass and colleagues toward providing evidence both of a meaningful unconscious and primary process mentation as a distinct mode of mentation. A few specific references are: Shevrin, Bond, Hertel, Williams, and Brakel 1992; Snodgrass, Shevrin, and Kopka, 1993; Shevrin, Bond, Brakel, Hertel, and Williams 1996; and Brakel 2004.

effects similar to those of the active drugs; and 2) there is an additional fourth group in the study whose members are monitored but get no treatment at all.[4] Ths is important because improvement may be due to a) regression to the mean as intense symptoms wax and wane; and b) the natural course of many symptoms to fade and disappear over time; this improvement caused neither by any active agent or placebo.

Findings over many decades, in hundreds of experiments, on many types of ailments have shown that around one-third of subjects receiving placebo treatments show some improvement, according to a review article by Asbjorn Hrobjartsson and Peter Gotzche (2001, p.1594). In addition, over these decades several different hypotheses concerning the mechanisms for the placebo response have been proposed. (For this history see Arthur Shapiro and Louis Morris 1978; Irving Kirsch 2004; and Steve Stewart-Williams and John Podd 2004.)

One of the first explanations proposed was based on personality, specifically that those who did well on placebos were characterologically more suggestible (Henry Beecher, 1955). Although this is a plausible hypothesis, several subsequent studies (reviewed in Shapiro and Morris 1978, pp.374–376) demonstrated that placebo effects varied quite independently of personality type, with suggestible subjects showing no increased placebo effect overall.

Another explanation concerns conscious expectancy. There have been many experiments showing that *conscious* expectation of an improvement with a particular treatment does have a pronounced effect on outcome. (See Stewart-Williams and Podd 2004 for references.) One of the clearest examples is a study done by Martina Amanzio, Antonella Pollo, Guiliano Maggi, and Fabrizio Benedetti (2001, p.205) in which they found that 'hidden injections were significantly less effective...compared with open injections (in full view of the subject)' in achieving pain relief.[5] On the other hand, it has been argued that expectations cannot play much of a role in double-*blind* studies; but note that even subjects in a double blind placebo study may believe that they will get the active drug and they will therefore get better.

Despite this, there is at least one very interesting study (Lee Park and Lino Covi 1965) with findings that call into question the relation between belief in

---

[4] Even this group does receive some professional care and attention and is therefore different from the unmonitored natural case.

[5] The very title of a recent article by Benedetti and his colleagues (F. Bendetti, C. Arduino, S. Costa, S. Vighetti, L. Tarenzi, I. Rainero, and G. Asteggiano 2009) indicates the importance of expectancy. The publication is titled: 'Loss of expectation-related mechanisms in Alzheimer's disease makes analgesic therapies less effective.'

the active drug's efficacy and symptomatic improvement. In the Park and Covi (1965) study, 14 patients received and were told that they were receiving placebo rather than an active medication. Fully 6 of those still felt they were getting the active drug, no matter what they were informed. Those 6 patients *and* the 8 patients who believed they were receiving just a placebo all showed significant improvement, with no significant differences between these two groups. Now there were obvious limits to this study: the evaluators of pre- and post-experiment symptoms were not blind as to the beliefs of the patients, and the number of patients was small. Nonetheless, results such as these suggest that expectation, especially conscious expectation, is at best just part of the picture. As I illustrate forthwith, robust placebo findings with animal subjects, where conscious expectations (at least the type humans have) cannot be playing the same role, strongly indicate that something operating outside of consciousness contributes to placebo responses.

Animal results: The role of conditioning in the placebo effect

It is commonly held that non-human animals do not have the same sorts of conscious expectations as do humans regarding the beneficial effects of medical treatments. Thus the placebo results obtained with animal subjects are very striking. Robert Ader and colleagues did many experiments demonstrating placebo effects as a result of conditioning. One in particular (reported in Ader 1988, pp.51–55) involves laboratory mice with induced systemic lupus erythematosus (SLE), an experimental model of systemic lupus erythematosus, a disease that is marked by organ-damaging autoimmune reactions. The experiment took place in two phases. In phase one, the mice in the group of interest were given a potent immunosuppressive drug with known deleterious side effects. The drug was given in a divided dose: first, it was injected paired with orally administered saccharine; next, the injected drug was given alone, with an oral administration of saccharine following later. Immunosuppressive effects were noted, but as predicted, they were incomplete, as more of the drug would be needed for better control of the disease. In the second phase of the experiment this same group of mice was split into three groups. Group A mice received a second injected dose of the immunosuppressive drug paired with saccharine, followed by more saccharine. Group B mice received a placebo injection paired with saccharine, followed by more saccharine. Note that this sequence—placebo injection paired with saccharine followed by oral saccharine—was designed to replicate the first phase of the experiment in order to see if the Group B mice could develop a conditioned immunosuppressive response to the placebo injection. Group C mice received no further treatment after phase one.

The results were as follows: Group C mice showed no further immunosuppression and no further improvement. Mice in Groups A and B, showed continued immunosuppresion and considerable improvement in their pathology. Most notably there were no significant differences in the improvements in mice in Groups A and B, despite the fact that Group B mice received just half as much of the dangerous drug. (Recall that Group B mice received the active drug only in phase one; in phase two of the experiment they were injected with a placebo.) The researchers concluded that Group B mice showed this robust placebo effect because of strong conditioned responses to the placebo injection.[6]

Implicit expectancy and the placebo effect

There is no reason to assume that placebo responses derive from single causes. Thus conditioning effects and conscious expectancy effects can be synergistic in facilitating placebo responses. (See Stewart-Williams and Podd 2004.) This is true also of non-conscious learning effects and implicit expectancy, both of which can also contribute to placebo responses, as can be readily appreciated in the following examples from Daniel Moerman and Wayne Jonas (2002, p.472). Two tablets are experienced as more effective than one; branded pills produce more placebo response than unbranded; and various colors of pills can produce differential effects. Further, Moerman (2002, p.81) discusses the profound effect that doctors' attitudes have on patient responses. A firmer diagnosis, with the physician expressing his/her expectation for improvement, did significantly improve patient symptom report whether or not any prescription was given. Physicians' conscious and expressed expectations make up part of the implicit expectations of patients, as do various non-consciously learned 'facts' concerning number, color, and product branding.

Transference and the placebo effect

Although not discussed very much as such in the literature on placebo responses (an exception is Shapiro and Morris 1978, p.391), the mechanism of

---

[6] See also Joel Dehasse's (1997) article on feline urinary spraying. Here Dehasse obtained similar conditioned placebo improvements after, and in addition to, initial responses to an active agent. This report helps to establish the generalizability of the Ader findings because Dehasse's work took place in a clinical setting (rather than an experimental one), with a natural, rather than induced symptom, and in cats instead of laboratory mice.

transference obviously plays a large role in the placebo effect.[7] If doctors' attitudes toward patients, both explicit and implicit, can produce placebo effects, we should expect that patients' positive reactions to doctors, both conscious and unconscious, would have an even greater impact.

Further, not only do people have specific transferences to specific doctors, there are general transferences to care-giving individuals as a class; transferences to doctors, not just to Dr. X or Dr. Y, and likewise to other health professionals. Similarly, people have general transferential attitudes toward procedures, medical equipment, therapeutic regimes, and to medications of all sorts, as well as particular transferences to each of these, which can be different at different times. In addition, people have transferences to self-care, and to themselves in sickness and then in health.

Finally, there are earlier more global background transferences, those allowing feelings of trust and wellbeing with other people. Probably stemming from nurturance, protection, and care, it is possible that domesticated animals have these sorts of basic positive transferential attitudes toward care-taking people too. In any case, at least in humans, to the extent that these various and complex transferences lead patients to 1) anticipate getting well, 2) regard the doctor as knowledgeable, and 3) feel well cared for and trusting in the doctor— all of these contribute to the placebo effect.

Transference, conditioning, and implicit expectations: All are primary process mediators of placebo effects

It should be of no embarrassment to psychoanalysts that transferences of various sorts, expectations of symptom amelioration (implicit and explicit), nonconscious learning, and some degree of (unconscious) conditioning, all produce placebo effects that account for *some* of the improvement reported in good psychoanalyses. After all as Moerman (2002, p.103) points out for therapeutics generally, 'In all likelihood, highly effective specific [regular active]

---

[7] Transferences are psychological attitudes, largely unconscious, that originate with key people in a person's past, particularly the parents, but also siblings, aunts and uncles, doctors, and teachers. These attitudes, often very emotionally charged (both positively and negatively) are called transferences when they are attributed (i.e., transferred) to current day figures who may bear only functional or superficial similarities to the original figures. The attribution to others, as well as the attitude itself, often occurs outside of consciousness. So a man with a nasty, authoritarian, hot-headed father may experience an older male boss as an angry autocrat, even if the boss is rather even tempered and studiously even handed. Note that transferences need not always be so far off the mark; people can also attribute (transfer) old attitudes to new people who do share essential qualities with the original figures, perhaps heightening the intensity of feelings.

treatment effects can be amplified (or damped down)...' by placebo effects. Put more strongly, it is a plausible claim that non-specific (placebo-type) responsiveness provides the underlying foundation necessary for every effective active agent, including those as diverse as successful surgery, pain relief, and psychoanalysis.

However, that is not the only relationship between psychoanalysis and the placebo effect. An aspect of psychoanalytic theory—specifically the formal operating principles of primary process mentation[8]—can help explain some of the basic psychological mechanisms contributing to the placebo response. Let us first take up conditioning and the primary process mechanisms of condensation and displacement. In classical Pavlovian conditioning the *unconditioned response*, e.g., salivating when food is present, is conditioned to take place when there is a bell sound but *no food*, at which point the salivating is a *conditioned response*. The creation of such a conditioned response can occur only after a number of trials when food follows immediately after the bell sound, i.e., the bell sound and the food following it are paired. One can appreciate then that first there is a *condensation*—responses to the contiguous bell *plus* food; and then a *displacement*—responses to the bell alone, the *bell standing for food coming*. The study described involving mice with experimentally induced SLE, although more complex, operates on the same classical conditioning and primary process principles.[9]

A different formal aspect of primary process mentation helps explain the implicit expectancies and some facets of non-conscious learning contributing to the placebo effect. Why is it that pills with brand names are reported as more effective than those without? Why does the color of a pill matter? For that matter, why do drug companies spend millions in advertising dollars and hours of brain-storming in choosing product names for medications? Is this a rational activity for the drug companies? The answer is 'yes' because the category 'successful medication' is one far from solely constituted on the basis of rational principles, such as the drug's chemical structure and modes of action. In fact 'successful medication' is a category equally dependent upon doctors

---

[8] For a review of the formal operating principles of primary process mentation including condensation and displacement, and for more on the primary processes in general see the section on 'A-rationality: General considerations' in Chapter 3 of this volume. Those wanting a more complete understanding of primary process a-rationality, its relation to psychoanalytic theory, and in particular its overall standing with respect to the philosophy of mind and action should also see Brakel (2009).

[9] For more on primary process a-rationality and conditioning see the subsection on 'A-rationality in classical conditioning' in Chapter 3 of this volume.

and patients having positive associations concerning such a-rational matters as its brand, name, color, shape, etc., seemingly small and inessential aspects of the drug in question. These insignificant attributes figure prominently whenever categorizations are based on the primary process with its a-rational principles; and it is clear that such primary process categorizations underlie much of the implicit expectancy and non-conscious learning involved in placebo responses.[10]

Finally transference itself can be understood in formal primary process terms. Transferences entail *displacements*—taking attitudes, feeling states, etc., that belong with someone in the past and displacing them onto someone in the present. In addition, there are also the primary process categorizations entailed in transferences. These mechanisms often come together when there is a displacement of a feeling or attitude attributed to a present-day person on the basis of some superficial, rather than essential or fundamental, similarity.

For an example relevant to the placebo effect, imagine a patient with a history of a painful illness early in childhood. Suppose that this patient was seen by three doctors, but experienced no improvement of symptoms until the third doctor, owing only to the natural course of the illness rather than any extraordinary medical activities. Suppose further that all three physicians had physical and/or emotional characteristics notable to the child at the time, but not remembered in adulthood. For instance, suppose the last doctor was a distracted pale red-headed woman, the first one a warm bald man with a beard, and the second doctor a funny tall African-American man. Is it not likely (or at least plausible) that a more positive transference will form toward doctors (and people) with some of the 'successful' physician's superficial primary process-type characteristics? Or, changing the example, imagine that the first doctor was a specialist who had to perform a painful procedure in order to effect a cure, but that the child's subsequent dramatic symptomatic improvement took place while under the care of a second physician, seen only briefly until the third doctor took over. Would we not have predictions about both positive and negative transferences, again predicated on rather inessential features of these three doctors?

---

[10] For a fuller discussion of the significance of inessential, superficial features in primary process mentation and categorizations see S. Freud 1900, p.597; 1901, p.278; 1905, pp.88–89; David Rapaport 1951a, pp.395,398; 1951b, p.708; Brakel 2004, pp.1134–1135; Brakel and Shevrin 2005, pp.1679–1680; and the subsection on 'A-rational categorizations in Chapter 3 of this volume.)

Conclusion

Like many medical treatments, a successful psychoanalysis might owe some portion of its good outcome to placebo effects. This is not a particularly remarkable fact. More interesting is that aspects of psychoanalytic theory—those pertaining to the formal workings of primary process mentation—can help explain some of the basic psychological mechanisms that underlie the placebo effect. The primary process categorizations predicated on inessential features and the primary process operation of displacement and condensation seem to function centrally in conditioning, unconscious learning, the formation of implicit expectancies, and transferences of all sorts. To the extent that these are indeed the mechanisms of the placebo effect, understanding psychoanalytic theory as it pertains to formal primary process mentation can help in the explanation of this most enigmatic phenomenon.

References

Ader, R (1988). The placebo effect and conditioned response. In R Ader, ed. *Experimental Foundations of Behavioral Medicine: Conditioning Approaches*, 47–66. Hillsdale NJ, Lawrence Erlbaum Assoc.

Amanzio, M, Pollo, A, Maggi, G, and Benedetti, F. (2001). Response variability to analgesics. *Pain*, **90**, 205–215.

Beecher, H (1955). The powerful placebo. *Journal of the American Medical Association*, **159**, 1602–1606.

Benedetti, F, Arduino, C, Costa, S, Vighetti, S, Tarenzi, L, Rainero, I, and Asteggiano, G (2009). Loss of expectation-related mechanisms in Alzheimer's disease makes analgesic therapies less effective. *Pain*, **121**, 133–144.

Brakel, LAW (2004). The Psychoanalytic assumption of the primary process: extra-psychoanalytic evidence and findings. *Journal of the American Psychoanalytic Association*, **52**, 1131–1161.

Brakel, LAW (2009). *Philosophy, Psychoanalysis, and the A-Rational Mind*. Oxford, Oxford University Press.

Brakel, LAW and Shevrin, H (2005). Anxiety, attributional thinking and the primary process. *International Journal of Psychoanalysis*, **86**, 1679–1693.

Dehasse, J (1997). Feline urine spraying. *Applied Animal Behavior Science*, **52**, 365–371.

Edelson, M (1984). *Hypothesis and Evidence in Psychoanalysis*. Chicago and London, The University of Chicago Press.

Freud, S (1900). *The Interpretation of Dreams*. Standard Edition, vols. 4 & 5. Trans. and ed. J Strachey. London, 1953, Hogarth Press.

Freud, S (1901). *The Psychopatholgoy of Everyday Life*. Standard Edition, vol.6. Trans. and ed. J Strachey. London, 1953, Hogarth Press.

Freud, S (1905). *Jokes and Their Relation to the Unconscious*. Standard Edition, vol. 8. Trans. and ed. J Strachey. London, 1953, Hogarth Press.

Grunbaum, A (1977). How scientific is psychoanalysis. In R.Stern, ed. *Science and Psychotherapy*, 219–254. New York, Haven Press.

Grunbaum, A (1981). The placebo concept. *Behavior Research and Therapy*, **19**, 157–167.

Grunbaum, A (1982). Can psychoanalytic theory be cogently tested 'on the couch? Part 1 & 2. *Psychoanalysis and Contemporary Thought*, **5**, 155–255, and 311–436.

Hrobjartsson, A and Gotzche, P (2001). Is the placebo powerless? *The New England Journal of Medicine*, **344**, 1594–1630.

Kirsch, I (2004). Conditoning, expectancy, and the placebo effect: Comment on Sterwart-Williams and Podd (2004). *Psychological Bulletin*, **130**, 341–343.

Moerman, D (2002). Explanatory mechanisms for placebo effects: cultural influences and the meaning response. In H Guess, A Kleinman, J Kusek, and L Engel, eds. *The Science of the Placebo: Toward an Interdisciplinary Research Agenda*, Chapter 4, 77–107, London, BMJ Books.

Moerman, D and Wayne, J (2002). Deconstructing the placebo effect and finding the meaning response. *Annals of Internal Medicine*, **136**, 471–476.

Park, L and Covi, L (1965). Nonblind placebo trial. *Archives of General Psychiatry*, **12**, 336–345.

Rapaport, D (1951a). States of consciousness. In M Gill, ed. *The Collected Papers of David Rapaport*, 385–404, New York, Basic Books.

Rapaport, D (1951b). Toward a theory of thinking. In D Rapaport, ed. *Organization and Pathology of Thought*, 689–730. New York, Columbia University Press.

Shevrin, H, Bond J, Hertel, R, Marshall, R,Williams, W, and Brakel, LAW (1992). Event-related potential indicators of the dynamic unconscious. *Consciousness and Cognition*, **1**, 340–366.

Shevrin, H, Bond, J, Brakel, LAW, Hertel, R, and Williams, W (1996). *Conscious and Unconscious Processes: Psychodynamic, Cognitive, and Neurophysiologic Convergences*. New York, Guilford Press.

Snodgrass, M, Shevrin, H, and Kopka, M (1993). The mediation of intentional Judgments by unconscious perceptions: The influences of task strategy, task preference, word meaning, and motivation. *Consciousness and Cognition*, **2**, 194–203.

Shapiro, A and Morris, L (1978). The placebo effect in medical and psychological therapies. In S Garfield and A Bergin, eds. *Handbook of Psychotherapy and Behavior Change* (2nd Edition), 369–410. New York, Wiley.

Stewart-William, S and Podd, J (2004). The placebo effect: dissolving the expectancy vs. conditioning debate. *Psychological Bulletin*, **130**, 324–340.

Part VI

Explanations and conclusions

Philosophy of science

Chapter 6

Explanations and conclusions

This book presents a number of problems located in a borderland between philosophical investigations and psychoanalytic theory. It has been my belief that since this border zone ought to be interesting, available, congenial, and at the same time challenging to both disciplines, problematic puzzles would be best solved using methods from each of them as well as tools common to both. Philosophers and psychoanalysts (theorists and clinicians alike) seek explanations for all manner of situations producing '…a psychological feeling of puzzlement [that] gives rise to a demand for explanation' (Sherwood 1969, p.14).

A therapeutic psychoanalysis, for example, can be conceptualized as a series of explanations of a patient's seemingly irrational behaviors and mental states. These explanations rely on a complex combination of uncovering past attitudes and concerns, along with inferences about the patient's current unconscious mental processes, such that patients can ultimately be better understood by their analysts, other people, and most importantly by the patients themselves. While this sort of clinical psychoanalytic explanation is not the type of explanation highlighted in the current volume, it does figure in all of the clinical psychoanalytic material presented in every chapter: in the psychoanalytic cases briefly presented in the chapter on agency (Chapter 4), in the lengthier case reported in the unconscious knowing chapter (Chapter 2), and in the many psychoanalytic examples offered as illustrative in the chapter on vagueness (Chapter 3).

With these clinical explanations in the background, in this the final chapter, in addition to offering summaries and conclusions, I examine the other sorts of explanations that each of the chapters has provided. Chapters 2–4, with respect to their explanatory aims, are more modest than Chapter 5. Hence I deal with them relatively briefly. Chapter 5, on the other hand, has a more ambitious explanatory goal. Therefore, I explore the nature of the explanation proposed in that chapter in much greater detail.

Explanations: Chapters 2–4

The sorts of explanations that have been central in this book are philosophical and/or scientific in nature. Most straightforward is the discussion in Chapter 2,

'Unconscious knowing: Psychoanalytic evidence in support of a radical epistemic view.' This chapter aims to strengthen the radical epistemological position that more can be understood (and explained) if we take knowledge to be prior to belief, both conceptually and ontologically. How is strength gained for the 'knowledge-first' account? Chapter 2 achieves this by providing a first-line type of explanation—empirical evidential support *for* the radical view, and *against* the opposing view. In this case the supporting evidence consists in research findings based on different experimental paradigms, all having psychoanalytically relevant data and methods. Indeed, while none of these findings can definitively prove the claims of the radical view, all of them taken together weigh heavily in favor of 'knowledge-first' explanations. Why? Because there is the combined and convergent evidence of several different types of empirical cases, each of which by inference to the best explanation[1] supports the 'knowledge-first' position over that of 'belief-first.'

Chapter 3, 'The limits of rationality: Vagueness, a case study' presents the discovery of a strange phenomenon: In attempts to deal with vagueness (vague concepts, vague properties, ontic vagueness, etc.), all with impeccable rationality, many and diverse philosophical accounts look surprisingly a-rational; i.e., analogous to the sorts of primary process-based thinking met with in psycho-analytic clinical practice, in the mentation of young children, in psychosis, and in dream reports. The explanation for this, while it seems simple, might in fact be profound: namely, that a-rationality emerges because it is a large and inevitable part of the way we think. This leads to more speculative metaphysical notions. First, it becomes possible to accord ontic vagueness along with a-rational objects[2] the same status as regular objects. Further, the ubiquitous presence of a-rational/primary process mentation as part of our ongoing cognitive processes introduces the possibility that the world is structured in such a way that these a-rational concepts, alongside the rational ones, play a vital role in helping us capture (or imagine) the actual (mind-independent) nature of the world.

Chapter 4, 'Agency: "me"-ness in action' proposes explanatory answers for both a philosophical problem and a psychoanalytic one, by the use of analogy. The chapter begins with the view that despite the wide use of a variety of other terms and diagnostic labels, a central (perhaps *the* central) problem in many (most) psychoanalytic patients involves conflicts about agency. After illustrating

---

[1] Much more will be said about 'inference to the best explanation' later in this chapter.

[2] What I have termed 'a-rational objects' are discussed at length in Chapter 3 of this volume. (See also Brakel 2009, Chapter 3.)

this point with a number of cases, I leave the psychoanalytic domain (temporarily) to investigate the fascinating philosophical problem of what 'me' I care about when I am concerned with my own survival. What I find is a surprise. Reviewing various thought experiments, and the strengths and weaknesses of the philosophical accounts they evoke, I propose that the answer to the philosophical problem is analogous to that in the psychoanalytic situation: It is my *agency* that is the 'me' with which I am concerned when I am concerned about my own survival. With agency now at the center both for psychoanalytic patients and in the philosophical dilemma concerning one's own survival, I complete my own account of agency as one that is necessarily 1) singular, 2) involves a willingness-to-act, and 3) is marked by actions for which 'why' questions, either at a psychological or biological/evolutionary level, have application.

The virtues of analogy as part of a good explanation are recognized by David Lewis (1986/1993, p.187) and are even more resoundingly endorsed by Paul Thagard (1978, pp. 89–91), who says '…analogy between phenomena… *improves* [his emphasis] the explanations…because…we get increased understanding of one set of phenomena if the kind of explanation used…is similar to ones already used' (p.91). In the agency chapter it is not clear that either set of phenomena is sufficiently well established or well explained such that the other would be the clear beneficiary of an explanation based on analogy. On the other hand, the analogy between the role of agency as the 'me' we care about when we care about our survival, and that of agency in psychoanalytic work points toward a unified conceptualization about agency in both fields.

Regarding Chapter 5, notwithstanding the simplicity suggested by its title, 'The placebo effect: Psychoanalytic theory can help explain the phenomenon,' the actual nature of the explanation provided is rather complex. This is the case despite the fact that I have claimed (rather boldly) that placebo occurrences can be explained (at least partly) on the basis of two better-known phenomena—positive conditioning and positive transference.[3] Certainly this is not a deductive explanation. However, beyond that, just what sort of explanation is this? I will take this up in the section to follow.

---

[3] 'Positive' conditioning in the context of Chapter 5 and the current chapter is meant to indicate conditioning that increases a therapeutic response. 'Positive' with respect to transference refers to those transferences of good feelings including being well cared for, protected, loved, loving, etc.

Explanations: Chapter 5

Does Chapter 5 offer a philosophical analysis?

There is the possibility that understanding the placebo effect in terms of positive conditioning and positive transference phenomena really is more of a philosophical analysis than a scientific explanation. Bas van Fraassen (1987) states:

> If philosophy is the removal of wonder, as Aristotle said, its proper enterprise is explanation. And producing, elaborating, defending the best explanations you can—providing possible ways of understanding, seeing how things could have been the way they are—is philosophy (p.259).

Now, van Fraassen is not headed where I wish to go. Whereas I want to make clear the distinctions between philosophical analyses and scientific explanations, van Fraassen's article discusses the problems associated with thinking that successful explanations are true.[4] However, van Fraassen's evocative phrase characterizing philosophy as 'explaining how things could be the way they *are*' lends itself to a contrast with science, where (most) explanations are not about the plausible and imaginable, but instead about how things *are caused*, and how *this* rather than *that* happens and then why.

In his article 'What is a philosophical analysis?,' Jeffrey King (1998, pp.155–179) presents (but then does not fully agree with) the classical view that philosophical analyses are conceptual analyses,[5] essentially aiming to determine what is constitutive of a particular concept. With concepts such as bachelor, the concept or property[6] of 'bachelor' is equivalent to its constituent parts—adult, never-married, male human being—and can be analyzed as such. Thus 'X is a bachelor if X is an adult, never-married, male human being' constitutes a philosophical analysis of the concept 'bachelor.' On the contrary 'X is a bachelor if X is a bachelor' is not a philosophical analysis of the concept 'bachelor' even though 'bachelor' is equivalent to 'bachelor' because there is no consideration of the concept's constituent parts.

---

[4] This is in keeping with van Fraassen's strong views of explanation as pragmatic and context dependent.

[5] For King, the differences between philosophical and scientific analyses are not rigidly distinct. Instead for King this distinction is determined by '...the sort of epistemic relations typical members of the linguistic community bear to the analyzed property' (p.169); or to put it bluntly whether philosophers or scientists are the parties interested in the explanations.

[6] On King's account the analyses of concepts need not be distinct from the analyses of properties.

Ernest Sosa's (1983) view of philosophical analysis is quite similar to this. It is the, 'description of the logical constitution of an object of analysis (an analysandum) by providing a property (an analysans) that reveals such constitution…by specifying a set of constituents of the analysandum and specifying further how those constituents constitute it' (p.700). A philosophical analysis can disambiguate certain epistemologic/ontologic confusions. For example (Sosa 1983, p.695), a person may be thinking of a cube without knowing that he/she is thinking of something that is necessarily a closed solid with six square sides. A philosophical analysis makes epistemologically accessible the ontologic constituents—in this case, the ontological constituents of cubes.

So by these criteria, does characterizing the placebo effect as a phenomenon involving positive conditioning and positive transference constitute a philosophical analysis? I think not. First, unlike the situation with cubes and closed solids with six square sides where every instance of the latter is an instance of the former, there are many positive transferences and positive conditionings that have nothing whatsoever to do with the placebo effect. Thus even if this were a philosophical analysis, in so far as it does not specifically differentiate the placebo effect from other instances of positive transferences and conditionings, as it stands, it is either not a very good analysis or a very incomplete one.

What if we were to add other parts necessary to uniquely constitute the placebo effect, e.g., a symptom to be monitored, a treatment situation, a procedure to be administered, and perhaps some state of expectation? Despite this it appears problematic, but now in a different way. Now the difficulty is much the same as it would be were we to take the case, 'X is water if X is equal to H_2O,' to be characterized as a strictly philosophical analysis. Indeed, water *is* constituted by the properties of two hydrogen atoms and one of oxygen, and to know this is to make its ontological properties accessible epistemologically; and yet there is something more. There were scientific discoveries and explanations involved in understanding that this particular liquid (and water in its solid and gaseous forms) has the particular atomic configuration of two hydrogen atoms and one oxygen atom, yielding 'H_2O.' Whereas the concept 'bachelor' means the same thing as its constitutive parts 'never-married, adult, human male,' and that is all there is to it; knowing the constitutive parts of 'water' as the properties of the molecule 'H_2O' reveals more than just an equivalence of meaning. The placebo effect as constituted by positive conditioning and transference more resembles the water/H_2O case, as there are scientific hypotheses and explanations involved, not merely definitions.

However, although we can conclude that Chapter 5 offers a scientific rather than a philosophical analysis of the placebo effect, there are clear differences between the scientific explanation of 'water' as 'H_2O'and that of the proposed explanation for the placebo effect. Thus, whereas one can deduce every time the fact that 'H_2O'—the molecular configuration of two atoms of hydrogen to one of oxygen—will fully, completely, and uniquely constitute 'water'; there is no way to deduce 'the placebo effect' given the combination of positive conditioning and positive transference, and whatever other parts we may add, in any configuration. Indeed, the explanation I proposed for the placebo effect is not a deductive one. Thus, after briefly presenting some general criteria for scientific explanations (both deductive and non-deductive) in the subsection just below, I return to a more specific version of the question: just what sort of *scientific* explanation does Chapter 5 provide?

General and basic criteria of scientific explanations

To the extent that scientifically devised medicines are the effective agents in symptom reduction, sugar pills, and other non-specifically active treatments[7] would not be expected to produce any symptomatic improvements. However, surprisingly in roughly one-third of trials in countless and diverse situations, placebo-based symptom amelioration occurs. Two related but distinct questions arise immediately: 1) How can the placebo phenomenon be explained? 2) What is it about the placebo phenomenon that we can explain? To begin to address both questions, let us turn to Robert Nozick's (1981, p.121) instructive discussion about the structure of scientific theories, in which he provides a framework for understanding what can and cannot (yet) be explained. He says, '...given that N is a natural or privileged state, why is it forces of type F, not of some other type F', that produce deviations from N?' So substituting for the variables, N, F, and F', in our current quest we get: given that no improvement would be the natural state following placebo administration (N), why is it that positive conditioning and positive transference (F), rather than some other processes (F'), produce significant increases over the expected natural state of nil improvement with placebos (change in N)? It should be evident that this is a question not yet answerable, at least in my opinion,

---

[7] I use the rather awkward phrase 'non-specifically active treatment' because placebos should be 'non-specifically active' rather than inert. In other words, in order for proper placebo versus agent-to-be-assessed tests, the placebo should be comparable to the actual agent in every way, save the specific therapeutic effects to be tested. This means that placebos should be active, and not inert with respect to side effects. Of course, the placebo agent should be administered just as is the actual one, and all the perceptible features should match. Aside from providing a fairer test, this allows participants to remain blind as to whether they are receiving placebo or the actual agent in their trials.

as I have not been able to propose alternative hypotheses for placebo-effect causes.

Instead, the work in Chapter 5 aims to address a more fundamental question, the answer to which can also reveal what we *can* explain about the placebo effect: 'Given that no improvement is the natural and expected state following placebo administration (N), *what* are the forces (F) operative producing the increase in symptom improvement (deviation in N)?' I have proposed that the forces at work driving the placebo effect are positive conditioning and positive transference. Although Nozick's question, 'Why these forces (F) and not others (F′)?,' remains unanswered, my proposal to understand which forces (F) drive the placebo effect and how they do so is a viable sort of explanation nonetheless.

Interestingly, Nozick would not dispute that the material in Chapter 5 counts as a scientific explanation. He maintains that 'Explanation proceeds by explaining some things in terms of others...' (1981, p.115). Peter Lipton (1990/1993, p.220) says something quite similar. In discussing non-deductive scientific theories in particular, he states that there is an 'obvious pragmatic' requirement for any good explanation namely that 'something new' must be gained.[8] Richard Boyd, also along the same lines, describes a particular aspect of scientific explanatory theories:

> An explanation for a particular phenomenon will typically draw upon the resources of some more general theory. It will appropriate the theoretical resources of the broader theory (entities, mechanisms, processes, causal powers, physical magnitudes, and so on), and it will employ, and often elaborate upon, these resources in describing how the phenomenon in question is caused (1985/1991, p.270).

To understand the placebo effect in terms of positive conditioning and transferences is to add something new. Further, conditioning and transference are clearly parts of broader more general theories.

Thus, despite its limitations, the non-deductive explanation for the placebo effect I proposed in Chapter 5 meets these basic and general standards for scientific explanation outlined above. But how will it do when more specific requirements are considered? Raimo Tuomela (1981), also commenting on the nature of non-deductive explanations in science, provides just such a

---

[8] Interestingly, the addition of something new could (should) be considered a requirement for philosophical analyses too. Recall the discussion above in which the true statement: 'a bachelor is a bachelor' does not count as philosophical analysis, whereas the true statement: 'a bachelor is a never-married, adult, male, human' does. Only the second statement is one about the constitution of the concept 'bachelor'; and only this statement adds something new.

specific criterion: 'An explanans [the explanation] should make the explanandum [that which is to be explained] nomically more expectable that the latter is by itself, and it should convey relevant information concerning the explanandum' (p.272). Placebo effects were likely unexpected when researchers first sought to test drugs using placebo control groups in their experiments. However, today placebo effects have been often observed and are expected. Indeed, they become even more expectable and *understandable* once they are inferred to result from instances of positive transference and/or positive conditioning. Why? Because the operations of these latter two processes are relatively well understood, thereby rendering the mechanisms of the placebo effect less opaque and mysterious. Further, giving explanations using causes or mechanisms does convey important information about the placebo effect (the explanandum), and in fact is a standard to which scientific explanations are held. According to Lipton, 'we explain phenomena by giving their causes or… we explain them by a giving a mechanism…' (1990/1993, p.207). What kind of cause or mechanism? David Lewis (1986/1993, p.195) suggests: 'A good explanation ought to show that the causal processes at work are of familiar kinds; or that they are analogous to familiar processes….' So far, so good for my proposed explanation.

However, although the explanation for the placebo effect offered in Chapter 5 can be considered a viable, non-deductive, scientific explanation, I still have not directly answered the question as to exactly what sort of scientific explanation it is. I will do this forthwith.

What sort of explanation? 'Inference to *an* explanation'

I want to continue with Lewis (1986/1993) to introduce another consideration, as well as to support the claims above: 'A good explanation ought to show that the explanandum event had to happen given the laws and the circumstances; or at least that it was highly probable, and could therefore have been expected if we had known enough ahead of time; or at least that it was less surprising than it may have seemed' (p.195). Clearly, the explanation I proposed for the placebo effect only fits in the last category. It is certainly not the case that a placebo response is a necessary outcome given a certain law and particular circumstances; nor is the placebo effect even highly probable. Instead we know and can predict the base rate of the placebo response at around 30%, a change from the 0% expected before placebo effects were observed, and this higher-than-expected base rate is less surprising because of the mechanisms I proposed to underlie placebo effects.

However, this assertion is not immune to challenges. A critic could maintain that the base rate of the placebo effect could be predicted and expected merely by repeated observations; that advancing any cause or mechanisms for the placebo effect adds nothing. However, I think this critic would be wrong. Observations are not explanations. To say 'we can see placebo effect mediated symptomatic improvements 30% of the time and therefore we expect them to occur 30% of the time' in no way explains *why* these ameliorations occur so much more than the 0% that would have been anticipated prior to such observations. On the other hand, to *infer* that placebo effects consist of positive transferences and positive conditionings (in some combination), both of which can lead to symptom relief in ways that *can* be clearly understood, is to explain *why* we expect that placebo induced improvements should be seen in 30% rather than 0% of the trials.

Put this way, the explanatory inference offered in Chapter 5 could be viewed as an example of a type of scientific explanation familiar under the descriptive term of art, 'inference to the best explanation.' And this is quite close. However, more modestly and more accurately, explaining placebo effects in terms of positive transferences and positive conditioning should be characterized as 'an inference to *an* explanation,' with potential to be an inference to the best explanation, if the explanation proposed is 1) tested and fares well and 2) proves the best of competing explanations. (See Lipton 1991, especially p.57.)

Testing the inference to an explanation

Returning to David Lewis' comments on the previous page, we can readily see once again that my inference to an explanation of the placebo effect in terms of positive conditioning and transference does not explain a necessary event following deductively from a universal law. Rather it is a type of statistical explanation, and a statistical explanation predicting low probability at that.[9] For Wesley Salmon, predicting low probability is not a problem; what is important is '...a *prior probability* of the occurrence to be explained, as well as one or more *posterior probabilities*. A crucial feature of the explanation will be the comparison between the prior and the posterior probabilities' (1984/1993, p.95). With this in mind, let us take up the first requirement toward becoming an inference to the *best* explanation—testing the explanation proposed in Chapter 5.

---

[9] A universal 'covering' law predicting necessary events, the so called 'deductive-nomological' explanation, is one of two types of explanations famously described by Carl Hempel (1962/1993). The other type, 'probablistc-statistical,' is also a law-based explanation, but it is based on inductive law, and for Hempel requires that particular phenomena arise with 'high logical, or inductive probability' (p.23). Wesley Salmon (1984/1993) takes issue with Hempel on this latter matter, asserting that 'high probability does not constitute a necessary condition for legitimate statistical explanations' (p.94).

This is not, in principle, difficult. We know that the prior probability of a placebo effect is around 30% for many different symptoms. Take a symptom that has shown the 30% response to placebo and a considerably larger rate of symptomatic improvement, say 80%, to a specifically active drug. Next, arrange to reduce the positive transference effects. This can be done readily by having a mean or indifferent person administer the treatment to all participants, i.e., both to the group getting the placebo drug as well as to those receiving the specifically active medication. Or have no human contact between participants and treatment providers and no human follow-up in both groups. Now the posterior probability of symptom relief should be well lower than 30% in the participants receiving the placebo, while those receiving the specifically active drug should show but a small change in the 80% experiencing improvement.[10]

Similarly, and this would be especially clear with the animal cases, reduce the positive conditioning. Conditioning of the type described in Chapter 5 requires a great deal of precision, so that ensuring that little conditioning occurs would be unproblematic. Again animals receiving the specifically active drug should have minimal change in their response rate, while the animals in the placebo group should now show a far reduced posterior probability of symptomatic improvement.[11] If in either of these cases the posterior probability of placebo response remains at the prior probability level of around 30%, my explanation that it is the mechanisms of positive transference and positive conditioning that drive the placebo effect will have been defeated.[12]

A further test of the positive conditioning and transference explanation can be constructed (following Woodward 2007, pp.74–75) in order to rule out another challenge for the inference to the explanation proposed. Suppose that

----

[10] Note that 'small change' rather than 'no change' is expected in the active drug group. This is due to the hypothesis that unconscious positive transference and implicit positive conditioning always make at least small (and sometimes sizeable) contributions to the symptomatic relief seen in response to specifically active agents too. (See Chapter 5.)

[11] Results would be less striking if there were other causal mechanisms in addition to positive transference and conditioning driving the placebo effect because these would still be in effect.

[12] Were this negative result for my explanation to obtain, one could plausibly conclude that the placebo effect is merely correlated with instances of positive transferences and positive conditioning. This could be due to some common cause both for the placebo effect and positive transference and conditioning, or for other more contingent reasons. For example take alcohol abuse and liver damage. If these were merely correlated, curtailing such alcohol use would not decrease the prevalence of liver disease. Whereas if alcohol consumption were causative, decreasing its over-use would reduce the incidence of liver pathology.

it is not the positive conditioning or transference *per se*, but some outcome (or other factor) concomitant with these mechanisms, that causes the placebo effect, e.g., an increase in positive affect including heightened feelings of pleasure and wellbeing. It should be possible to increase such affects while decreasing the positive conditioning and transferences. For example, food and other rewards increasing pleasure can be given in a context that does not allow positive conditioning. (Remember that it is quite easy to disrupt a conditioning situation.) With respect to increasing positive affects while decreasing the relevant positive transferences, the treatments could now be administered by someone who, while the antithesis of physicianly (and thereby not likely to draw doctor transferences), e.g., a comedian, is very pleasing and joy promoting. If, under these circumstances, the placebo rates do drop significantly, the positive transferences and conditioning explanation for the placebo effect will have gained some support; but if the rate remains at around 30% my explanation will have been defeated.

Contrastive explanation

Explanations are often (perhaps always) offered in particular contexts, and they always have explicit or implied contrasts. (See van Fraassen 1980/1993; Tuomela 1980; Lewis 1986/1993; Lipton 1990/1993, 1990.) My explanation for the placebo effect is an attempt to explain the following contrast: Why are there placebo improvements at a rate greater than the expectable 0%? However, it is not an attempt to explain why this rate is around 30% and not 45%, nor is it an attempt to explain why person X is a placebo responder and person Y is not. Nonetheless, contrasts such as these—natural follow-up questions to my proposed explanation—are, in principle, possible to explain.[13] This is important for evaluating the proposed explanation as an explanation because, as will be taken up in the next subsection, an explanation's ability to generate other answerable contrastive questions, counts in favor of its 'goodness.'

The inference to an explanation in Chapter 5 regarding the causal mechanisms of the placebo effect does generate other answerable contrastive questions, including some hypotheses and predictions. Turning to one of the contrasts mentioned just above—why person X is a placebo responder, while

---

[13] This is not the case for what Peter Railton (1981/1993, p.175) describes as 'genuine probabilistic explanation [in which] there are certain why-questions that simply do not have answers—questions as to why one probability rather than another was realized in a given case,' e.g., why a particular U^{238} atom decayed at a particular moment (p.164). Railton continues, 'If there were a reason why one probabilistic outcome of a chance process was realized rather than another, we would not be dealing with a chance process' (p.165). (See also Tuomela 1981, p. 285 and Lewis 1986/1993, p.197.)

person Y is not—my proposed explanation entails the following prediction: Person X is someone more likely to be effected by positive transferences and positive conditioning, than is Person Y. This in turn could be readily tested in various populations, followed by further investigations about other factors differentiating subjects like Person X and those like Person Y. These follow-up studies would be, for instance, neuroanatomical, or socio-geographical, in other words at a level different from the bio-psychological level of positive transferences and conditioning, inferred to be the causative mechanisms of the placebo effect. Let me explain further with an actual example.

There is, as it happens, very new neurophysiological research exploring exactly this question—why some people are big placebo responders compared with others. Andrew Leuchter, James McCracken, Aimee Hunter, Ian Cook, and Jonathan Alpert (2009) have found that different genetic patterns regulating certain neurotransmitters in the brain, specifically modulating brain monoaminergic tone, are related to different degrees of placebo responding. It would be very good for my explanation if the genetic differences also predicted differences in positive conditioning and positive transference outcomes, with the high placebo responders showing better capacities for positive conditioning and positive transference induction and maintenance.[14]

It is time to examine, as promised, other factors contributing to the potential goodness of explanations and to evaluate how good as an explanation, in particular, is the inference to an explanation advanced in Chapter 5.

Evaluating Chapter 5's inference to an explanation

Clearly, there is a serious weakness in the explanation for the placebo effect presented in Chapter 5. It is the fact that no rival explanations have been offered or even suggested. Thus the proposal that positive transferences and positive conditioning are underlying causal mechanisms for the placebo effect cannot be an inference to the *best* explanation, but only an inference to *an* explanation.

However, even as it stands, the explanation does have certain merits. As I have shown above, one of its most important assets is that it is testable. In addition there are several other characteristics important to a good explanation,

---

[14] One might ask why this explanation for high versus low placebo responders does not constitute a rival for my proposed explanation of the placebo effect. The answer is that this study does not in any way 'explain' the placebo effect and it did not set out to do so. It was designed to see if there were neurophysiologic markers of one group versus another. Even the positive findings of their study do nothing to explain the mechanisms underlying the placebo effect itself.

which the explanation in question does possess to some considerable degree. These characteristics are:

1) Explanatory power, including predictions with new data, and the capacity to generate new and related questions (See Laudin 1981/1991, p.233; Fine 1984/1991, p.261; Boyd 1985/1991, p.349; Lipton 1991, p.59; Gasper 1991, p.289; Trout 1991, p.605.)

2) Simplicity and internal coherence (See van Fraassen 1977/1991, p.326; Thagard 1978, p.85–89; Boyd 1985/1991, p.350; Kim 1987/1993, pp.234–235; Lipton 1991, p.59; Gasper 1991, p.289.)

3) Diversity of phenomena explained

4) Consilience and systematic organization, both with neighboring fields and disciplines with distant theories. (See Thagard 1978, p.79–85; Cartwright 1980/1991, p.380; Fine 1984/1991, p.261–262; Kim 1987/1993, pp.234–235; Lipton 1991, p.59; Trout 1991, p.608.)[15]

Using these four criteria, let us now examine how the explanation proposed in Chapter 5 stacks up. 1) Explanatory power: Chapter 5's inference to an explanation demonstrates considerable explanatory power both with respect to generating new and related research questions that directly follow, and in providing hypotheses to new data. 2) Simplicity: With regard to simplicity, the explanation for placebo presented in Chapter 5 posits a causal mechanism based on two better-known phenomena, backed up by a general theory in the case of positive transference, and a huge accumulation of empirical observations in the case of positive conditioning. The explanation itself is theoretically simple, with few moving parts. 3) Diversity: The best case for diversity of phenomena explained is to be made by noting the remarkable role that positive conditioning (and possibly positive transference) plays in mediating undeniable

---

[15] Interestingly, explanations in both philosophy of science and psychoanalysis suffer from the same conflict concerning internal coherence and systematic organization across diverse areas. In philosophy of science, there are those who feel that internal coherence and broad external organization are predictive of the truth of scientific explanations. For these philosophers, the scientific realists, there are just too many things admitting of consistent explanations for mere coincidence to obtain rather than (at least approximate) truth. Those embracing different forms of irrealism take issue with the proponents of scientific realism, arguing that theories can be consistent internally and give systematic organization across many domains and still not be even approximately true; but rather can merely reflect our own human cognitive way of organizing things.

Similarly, for psychoanalytic interpretations, there are some theorists who contend that there may be no consistent relation between truth (or approximate truth) and any understanding that the patient and analyst dyad construct. These analysts, adherents of the coherence theory of truth, are at odds with other analytic theorists who hold for a correspondence model of interpretation and truth.

and strong placebo effects in animals, much as these mechanisms work in the placebo effects reported by conscious, expectant adult human beings. 4) Consilience: The explanation that positive transference and positive conditioning are vital causal mechanisms in the placebo effect not only sheds light on a mysterious, albeit robust, phenomenon, but does so uniting data and theories across disciplines, generating questions answerable by findings from yet other domains. These are the strengths of the explanation offered in Chapter 5. These strengths bring back to mind the contributions of the other chapters, and of the book as a whole—all of which I will comment upon forthwith, very briefly, and finally.

Philosophy and psychoanalysis

The problems that philosophers pose in speculation are often problems that analysts meet with in practice. Explanations for the puzzles shared by both fields can best be solved by crossing the barriers between these disciplines, not only by using concepts, theories, mechanisms common to both, but also by giving application of the processes of one discipline to the data of the other.

***

It has been my great pleasure and privilege to work on this book. I am optimistic for the long-term survival, in exuberant good health, of the ever-fascinating and always-engaging interdisciplinary field of psycho-philosophical analysis. Although this work is at an end for now, I am already looking forward to future forays.

References

Boyd, R (1985/1991). Observations, explanatory power, and simplicity. In R Boyd, P Gaspers, and J Trout, eds. *The Philosophy of Science*, Chapter 19, 349–377. Cambridge Mass and London England, MIT Press.

Brakel, LAW (2009). *Philosophy, Psychoanalysis, and the A-Rational Mind.* Oxford, Oxford University Press.

Cartwright, N (1980/1991). The reality of causes in a world of instrumental laws. In R Boyd, P Gaspers, and J Trout, eds. *The Philosophy of Science*, Chapter 20, 379–386. Cambridge Mass and London England, MIT Press.

Fine, A (1984/1991). The natural ontological attitude. In R Boyd, P Gaspers, and J Trout, eds. *The Philosophy of Science*, Chapter 12, 261–277. Cambridge Mass and London England, MIT Press.

Gasper, P (1991). Causation and explanation: introductory essay. In R Boyd, P Gaspers, and J Trout, eds. *The Philosophy of Science*, 289–297. Cambridge Mass and London England, MIT Press.

Hempel, C (1962/1993). Explanations in science and history. In D-H Ruben, ed. *Explanation*, Chapter 1, 17–42. Oxford, Oxford University Press.

Kim, J (1987/1993). Explanatory realism, causal realism, and explanatory exclusion. In D-H Ruben, ed. *Explanation*, Chapter 9, 228–245. Oxford, Oxford University Press.

King, J (1998). What is a philosophical analysis? *Philosophical Studies*, **90**, 155–179.

Laudin, L (1981/1991). A confutation of convergent realism. In R Boyd, P Gaspers, and J Trout, eds. *The Philosophy of Science*, Chapter 12, 223–245. Cambridge Mass and London England, MIT Press.

Leuchter, A, McCracken, J, Hunter, A, Cook, I and Alpert, J (2009). Monamine Oxidase A and Catchol-O-Methyltransferease functional polymorphisms and the placebo response in major depressive disorder. *Journal of Clinical Psychopharmacology*, **29**, 372–377.

Lewis, D (1986/1993). Causal explanations. In D-H Ruben, ed. *Explanation*, Chapter 7, 182–206. Oxford, Oxford University Press.

Lipton, P (1990/1993). Contrastive explanation. In D-H Ruben, ed. *Explanation*, Chapter 8, 207–227. Oxford, Oxford University Press.

Lipton, P (1991). *Inference to the Best Explanation*. London and New York, Routledge Press.

Nozick, R (1981). *Philosophical Explanations*. Cambridge Mass, Harvard University Press.

Railton, P (1981/1993). Probabilities, explanation, information. In D-H Ruben, ed. *Explanation*, Chapter 6, 160–181. Oxford, Oxford University Press.

Salmon, W (1984/1993). Scientific explanations and the causal structure of the world. In D-H Ruben, ed. *Explanation*, Chapter 3, 78–112. Oxford, Oxford University Press.

Sherwood, M (1969). *The Logic of Explanation in Psychoanalysis*. New York and London, Academic Press.

Sosa, E (1983). Classical analysis. *The Journal of Philosophy*, **80**, 695–710.

Thagard, P (1978). The best explanation: criteria for theory choice. *The Journal of Philosophy*, **75**, 76–92.

Trout, JD (1991). The philosophy of psychology: introductory essay. In R Boyd, P Gaspers, and J Trout, eds. *The Philosophy of Science*, 605–614. Cambridge Mass and London England, MIT Press.

Tuomela, R (1980). Explaining explaining. *Ekenntnis*, **15**, 211–243.

Tuomela, R (1981). Inductive explanation. *Synthese*, **48**, 257–294.

van Fraassen, B (1977/1991). The pragmatics of explanation. In R Boyd, P Gaspers, and J Trout, eds. *The Philosophy of Science*, Chapter 17, 317–327. Cambridge Mass and London England, MIT Press.

van Fraassen, B (1980/1993). The pragmatics of explanation. In D-H Ruben, ed. *Explanation*, Chapter 11, 275–309. Oxford, Oxford University Press.

van Fraassen, B (1987). Armstrong on laws and probabilities. *Australasian Journal of Philosophy*, **65**, 243–60.

Woodward, J (2007). Causation with a human face. In H Price and R Corry, eds. *Causation, Physics, and the Constitution of Reality*, Chapter 4, 66–105. Oxford, Oxford University Press.

Name Index

Subject Index